Basic First Aid

National Safety Council

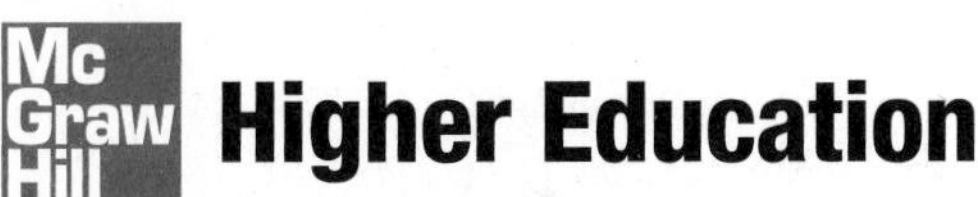

Boston Burr Ridge, IL Dubuque, IA Madison, WI New York
San Francisco St. Louis Bangkok Bogotá Caracas Kuala Lumpur
Lisbon London Madrid Mexico City Milan Montreal New Delhi
Santiago Seoul Singapore Sydney Taipei Toronto

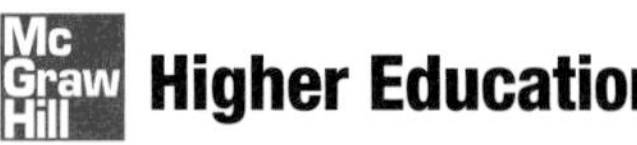

Higher Education

BASIC FIRST AID

Published by McGraw-Hill, a business unit of The McGraw-Hill Companies, Inc., 1221 Avenue of the Americas, New York, NY 10020.

This book is printed on acid-free paper.

3 4 5 6 7 8 9 0 KGP/KGP 0 9 8 7 6 5

ISBN 0–07–301673–x

Publisher: *David T. Culverwell*
Senior Sponsoring Editor: *Roxan Kinsey*
Developmental Editor: *Patricia Forrest*
Editorial Coordinator: *Connie Kuhl*
Outside Managing Editor: *Kelly Trakalo*
Outside Production Editor: *Marilyn Rothenberger*
Marketing Manager: *Lynn M. Kalb*
Senior Project Manager: *Sheila M. Frank*
Senior Production Supervisor: *Laura Fuller*
Lead Media Project Manager: *Audrey A. Reiter*
Media Technology Producer: *Janna Martin*
Senior Coordinator of Freelance Design: *Michelle D. Whitaker*
Cover/Interior Designer: *Seann Dwyer/Studio Montage, St. Louis, MO*
Lead Photo Research Coordinator: *Carrie K. Burger*
Photo Research: *Karen Pugliano*
Supplement Producer: *Brenda A. Ernzen*
Compositor and Art Studio: *Electronic Publishing Services Inc., NYC*
Typeface: *11.5/13 Minion*
Printer: *Quebecor World Kingsport*

Photo Credits: Figures 3.3, 3.4, 3.6, 3.7, 5.6: Courtesy Bradley R. Davis; Figures 3.5, 5.12, 7.3, 10.1a: © Mediscan; Figures 5.2, 5.3, 5.7: © Dr. P. Marazzi/Photo Researchers, Inc.; Figure 9.1a: Courtesy www.poison-ivy.org; Figure 9.1b: Courtesy M. D. Vaden, Certified; Arborist, Oregon; Figure 9.1c: © Gilbert Grant/Photo Researchers, Inc.; Figure 9.2a: Centers for Disease Control; Figure 9.2b: CDC/Harold G. Scott; Figure 9.4a: © Brad Mogen/Visuals Unlimited; Figure 9.4b: Photo by Scott Bauer, Agricultural Research Service, USDA; Figure 9.6: © DV13/Digital Vision/Getty; Figure 10.1b: © SIU/Visuals Unlimited; all other photographs © The McGraw-Hill Companies, Inc./Rick Brady, photographer.

Illustrations by Electronic Publishing Services Inc.: Jennifer Brumbaugh–3.14, 4.1, 8.1, 11.3;
Matthew McAdams–2.1, 3.1, 3.2, 3.11, 5.1, 7.2, 9.5, 10.3.

www.mhhe.com

About the National Safety Council

Founded in 1913, the National Safety Council (NSC) is a nonprofit membership organization devoted to protecting life and promoting health. Its mission "is to educate and influence society to adopt safety, health, and environmental policies, practices, and procedures that prevent and mitigate human suffering and economic losses arising from preventable causes."

The National Safety Council has been the leader in protecting life and promoting health in the workplace for over 90 years. The Council has helped make great improvements in workplace safety, and expanded their focus to include safety on the roads and in the home and community. Working through its 37,000 members, and in partnership with public agencies, private groups, and other associations, the Council serves as an impartial information gathering and distribution organization; it disseminates safety, health, and environmental materials from its Itasca, Illinois, headquarters through a network of regional offices, chapters, and training centers.

In 1990 NSC established First Aid and CPR courses to promote effective emergency response. Since then, they have grown to meet the changing needs of emergency responders at all levels of expertise. Upon successful completion of this course, you join more than 10 million National Safety Council trained responders protecting life and promoting health.

Acknowledgements

The National Safety Council wishes to thank the following Chapters and individuals for their assistance in developing this program:

For providing technical advice and assistance with photography: Safety Council of Maryland and Ms. Pat Raven, Director, Occupational Services, Safety Council of Maryland.

For providing technical advice and assistance with videotaping: the Arizona Chapter, National Safety Council, John Stubbs and C. J. Anderson.

For providing technical writing services: Tom Lochhaas, Editorial Services, Newburyport, MA.

For providing direction and support for National Safety Council Emergency Care programs: Donna M. Siegfried, Executive Director, Emergency Care & Home and Community Programs; Barbara Caracci, Director of Emergency Care Products and Training; Donna Fredenhagen, Manager of National Programs and Initiatives; Kathy Safranek, Project Administrator.

Publisher's Acknowledgements

Jason J. Goetz
Senior Safety Engineer
Worldwide Environmental, Health & Safety
Intel Corporation
Phoenix, AZ

Jeffrey Guy, M.D.
Director, Vanderbilt Regional Burn Center
Vanderbilt University Medical Center
Nashville, TN

James H. Howson
Director, Emergency Preparedness
New Jersey Hospital
Princeton, NJ

Debbie Kaye
Instructor, Dakota County Technical College
Minnesota Safety Council
Rosemont, MN

Tom Link
Safety and Health Council of North Carolina
Harrisburg, NC

Michael J. O'Brien
Education Coordinator
Emergency Medical Services
St. Vincent Hospital
Indianapolis, IN

Robb Rehberg, Ph.D.
Director and Chief, Emergency Medical Services
Montclair State University
Upper Montclair, NJ

Lisa Webb
Coordinator, Business Continuity & Disaster Recovery Planning
Delta Airlines

B. Drew Wellmon, D.O.
Wellmon Family Practice
Shippensburg, PA

Table of Contents

Chapter

1 Why Learn First Aid?

CHAPTER PREVIEW

- Need for First Aid Training
- What Is First Aid?
- Emergency Medical Services
- Be Prepared
- Legal Issues in First Aid
- Coping with a Traumatic Event

First aid training helps save lives. It's that simple. Whether on the job, in your home, or in the community, knowing first aid allows you to help someone who is injured or suddenly ill until help arrives or the person sees a healthcare provider.

In the United States every year:

- 2 million people are hospitalized because of injuries
- 140,000 die from injuries
- 500,000 die from heart attacks
- 150,000 die from strokes

You can help make a difference and maybe save a life.

In the workplace, over 1.5 million injuries happen every year that are serious enough to make the injured person miss work. Over 5000 workers die on the job from injuries. Figures 1-1 and 1-2 show the most common types of injuries and their causes. In many cases, if someone trained in first aid was present to give first aid, the results of the injury would be less severe or a life could be saved.

What Is First Aid?

First aid is the immediate help given to a victim of injury or sudden illness by a bystander until appropriate medical help arrives or the victim is seen by a healthcare provider. First aid is usually not all the treatment the person needs, but it helps the victim for the usually short time until advanced care begins.

Most first aid is fairly simple and does not require extensive training or equipment. With the first aid training in this course and a basic first aid kit, you can perform first aid.

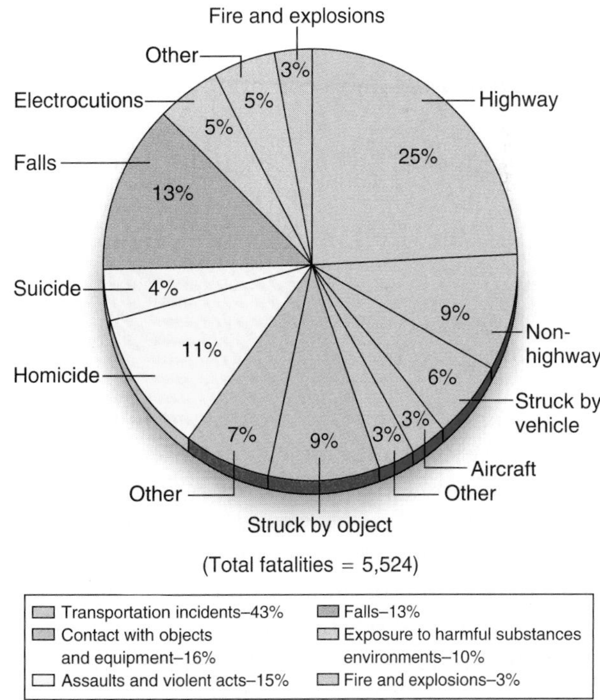

Figure 1-1 The manner in which workplace fatalities occurred. *Source:* U.S. Department of Labor, Bureau of Labor Statistics. Census of Fatal Occupational Injuries, 2002.

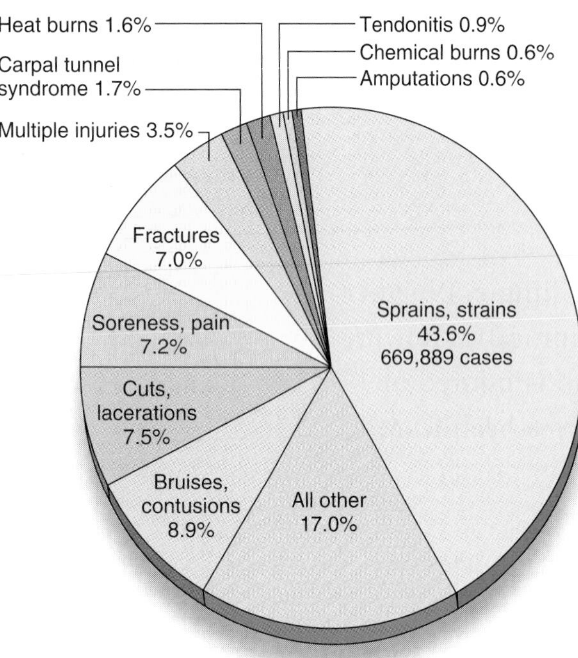

Figure 1-2 Occupational injuries and illnesses involving days away from work. *Source:* Bureau of Labor Statistics. U.S. Department of Labor, Survey of Occupational Injuries and Illnesses, 2001.

Goals of First Aid

- Keep the victim alive
- Prevent the victim's condition from getting worse
- Help promote recovery from the injury or illness
- Ensure the victim receives medical care

The Emergency Medical Services System

Workers and citizens who are trained in first aid are the first step in the Emergency Medical Services (EMS) system. As a first aider you are *only* the first step, so part of your responsibility is to make sure the EMS system responds to help a victim of injury or sudden illness by calling 911 (or your local or company emergency number). You will learn more about calling EMS in Chapter 2. In most communities in the United States, help will arrive within minutes. The first aid you give helps the victim until then.

Be Prepared

- ***Know what to do.*** This first aid course will teach you what to do.
- ***Stay ready.*** A first aid situation can occur anytime, anywhere. Think of yourself as a first aider who is always ready to step in and help. Other bystanders at the scene may feel helpless or hesitate to help, but you should feel confident that you can assist the victim.
- ***Have a personal first aid kit, and know where kits are in your workplace.*** Be sure first aid kits are well stocked with the right supplies. Keep emergency phone numbers, such as EMS, the Poison Control Center, and other emergency agencies, in a handy place.
- ***Know whether your community uses 911 or a different emergency telephone number.*** Note that this manual says "Call 911" throughout. If your community does not use the 911 system, call your local emergency number instead. Some companies have an internal emergency number you are expected to call, and that department will then call EMS.

Preventing Emergencies

Most injuries, and some sudden illnesses, can be prevented. This manual provides some prevention tips while you are learning first aid, but it is beyond the scope of this book to cover prevention in detail. You should follow these general guidelines for prevention:

- In the workplace, always follow safety procedures required by Occupational Safety and Health Administration (OSHA). If you have received safety training, use it. It takes only one lapse from a safety procedure to lose a life.

- In your home, take steps to prevent fires, accidental poisonings, and other injuries. Look for hazards and correct them.

Your First Aid Kit

Keep a well-stocked first aid kit in your home and vehicle, and know where one is kept at work. Take one with you on activities such as camping and boating. A cell phone is also helpful in most emergencies.

Make sure your first aid kit includes the items shown in Figure 1-3. Note that you may not necessarily use all items in a kit just because they are there. For example, first aiders do not give medications such as analgesics like aspirin or acetaminophen. However, some adult victims may choose to give themselves such medications.

Can You Be Sued for Giving First Aid?

Generally you do not need to be concerned about being sued for giving first aid. If you give first aid as you are trained in this course, and do your best, there is little chance of being found legally liable. To protect yourself it is recommended that you use the following guidelines:

1. Act ***only*** as you are trained to act.
2. Get a victim's consent before giving first aid.
3. Do not move a victim unnecessarily.
4. Call for professional help.
5. Keep giving care until help arrives.

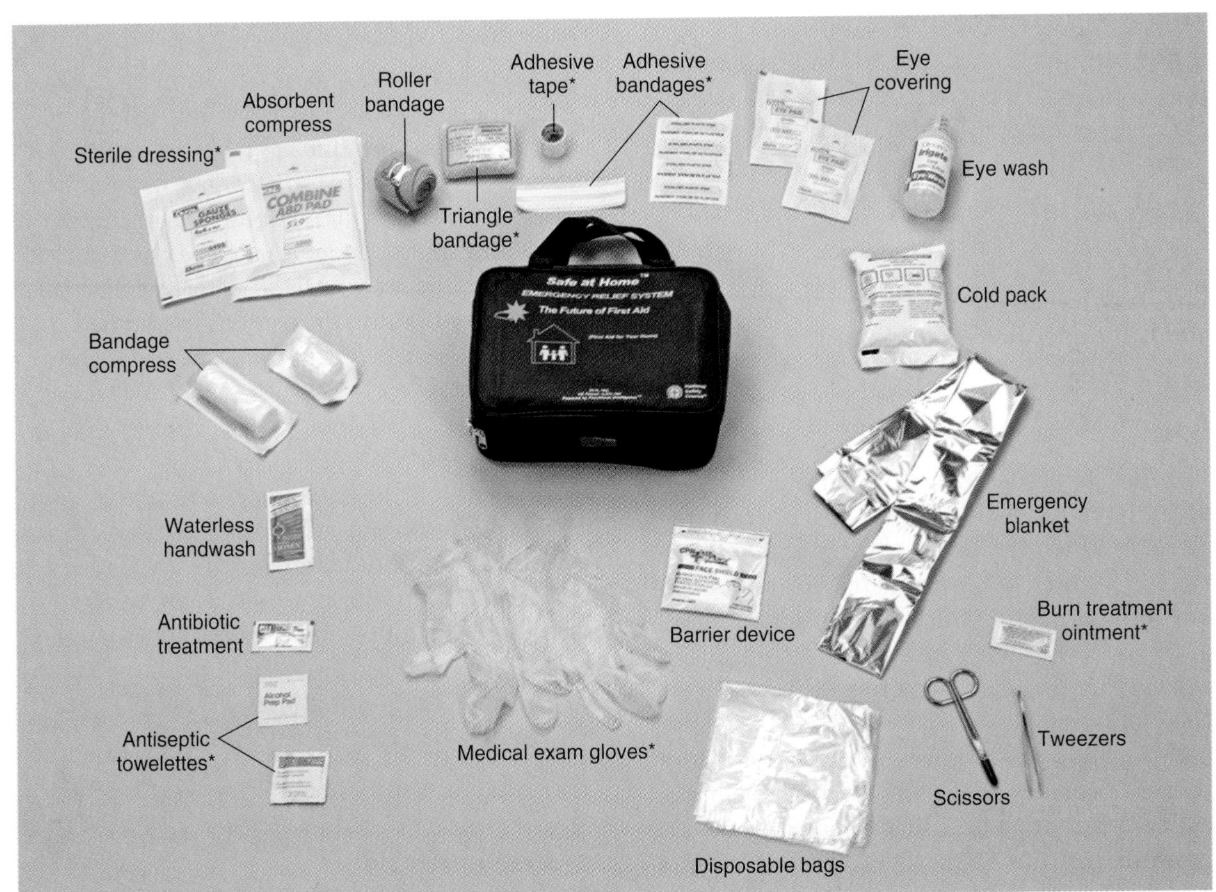

Figure 1-3 Components of a first aid kit (*denotes required item).

Learning Checkpoint 1

1. True or False: When you give first aid, the victim does not need to see a healthcare provider.

2. True or False: First aid given promptly can save lives and reduce severity of injuries.

3. Being prepared for an emergency means:

a. Knowing what to do

b. Being ready to act anytime, anywhere

c. Knowing how to get medical care for a victim

d. All of the above

Good Samaritan Laws

Most states have laws called **Good Samaritan laws** designed to encourage people to help others in an emergency without worrying about being sued. These laws protect you legally when you give first aid. It is unlikely you would be found liable or financially responsible for a victim's injury as long as you follow the guidelines mentioned on page 3. Ask your instructor about the specific Good Samaritan laws in your area.

Must You Give First Aid?

In most states you have no legal obligation to give first aid as a citizen or a bystander at the scene of an emergency. As the specific obligations may vary, ask your instructor about the law in your area. If you do begin giving first aid, however, you are obligated to continue giving care if you can and to remain with the victim.

Your job may require giving first aid, and that does make you legally obligated. This is called a **duty to act.** Off the job, however, depending on your state's laws, you are usually not legally required to give first aid except in special cases, such as parents or guardians caring for their child and other special situations.

Get the Victim's Consent

A responsive (awake and alert) victim must give consent before you can give first aid. Tell the person you have been trained and describe what you will do to help. The victim may give consent by telling you it is okay or by nodding agreement.

An unresponsive victim, however, is assumed to give consent for your help—this is called **implied consent.** Similarly, consent is assumed if a parent or guardian is not present and a child needs first aid.

Follow Standards of Care

Legally, you may be liable for the results of your actions if you do not follow accepted standards of care. **Standard of care** refers to what others with your same training would do in a similar situation. It is important you do only as you are trained. Any other actions could result in the injury or illness becoming worse.

You may be guilty of **negligence** if:

1. You have a duty to act
2. You breach that duty (by not acting or acting incorrectly)
3. Your actions or inaction causes injury or damages (including such things as physical injury or pain)

Examples of negligent actions could include moving a victim unnecessarily, doing something you have not been trained to do, or failing to give first aid as you have been trained.

Once you begin giving first aid, do not stop until another trained person takes over. Stay with the victim until help arrives or someone with equal or greater training takes over. If you leave the victim and the injury or illness becomes worse, this is called **abandonment.** Note that abandonment is different from justified instances of stopping care, such as if you are exhausted and unable to continue or you are in imminent danger because of hazards at the scene.

Coping with a Traumatic Event

Emergencies are stressful, especially when the victim does not survive. Not even medical professionals can save every victim. Injuries, illness, or circumstances are often beyond our control. After an emergency you may have a strong reaction, or later on you may have problems coping. This is normal—we are only human, after all. To help cope with the effects of this traumatic event:

- Talk to others: family members, coworkers, local emergency responders, or your family healthcare provider (without breaching confidentiality of the victim).
- Remind yourself your reaction is normal.
- Don't be afraid or reluctant to ask for professional help: Employee Assistance Programs and Member Assistance Programs can often provide such help.

Learning Checkpoint 2

1. True or False: Good Samaritan laws protect only professionals like paramedics and healthcare providers.

2. True or False: The best thing to do in any emergency is move the victim to your car and get him or her to an emergency room.

3. You have a duty to act when:

a. You stop at the scene of an emergency

b. You have taken a first aid course

c. You have a first aid kit with you

d. Your job requires you to give first aid when needed

4. Check off which victims you have consent to give first aid to:

_____ **a.** An unresponsive victim

_____ **b.** A child without parent or guardian present

_____ **c.** All victims, all of the time

_____ **d.** A victim who nods when you ask if it is okay to give first aid

_____ **e.** A child whose parent or guardian gives consent for the child

5. Check off things you should always do when giving first aid:

_____ **a.** Move the victim

_____ **b.** Do what you have been trained to do

_____ **c.** Try any first aid technique you have read or heard about

_____ **d.** Ask for victim's consent

_____ **e.** Stay with the victim until another trained person takes over

_____ **f.** Transport all victims to the emergency room in your vehicle

Chapter

2 Take Action in an Emergency

CHAPTER PREVIEW

- What You Can Do
- Avoiding Infectious Disease
- Assess the Victim
- Recovery Position

This chapter describes actions to take in all emergencies involving injury or illness. Always follow these basic steps:

1. Recognize the emergency and check the scene.
2. Decide to help.
3. Call 911 (when appropriate).
4. Check the victim.
5. Give first aid.
6. Seek medical attention (when appropriate).

Later chapters describe the specific first aid to give in different situations. This chapter describes the six steps above, how to protect yourself from infectious disease when giving first aid, and how to assess a victim.

What You Can Do

Follow these six steps in any emergency:

Recognize the Emergency and Check the Scene

You usually know there is an emergency when you see one. You see an injured or ill victim, or someone acting strangely. Or you may not see a victim at first but see signs that an emergency has occurred and that someone may be hurt.

Always check the scene when you recognize an emergency has occurred—before rushing in to help a victim. You must be safe yourself if you are to help another. Look for any hazards such as the following:

- Smoke, flames
- Spilled chemicals, vapors
- Downed electrical wires
- Risk of explosion, building collapse
- Roadside dangers, high-speed traffic
- Potential personal violence

If the scene is dangerous, ***stay away and call for help.*** Do not become a victim yourself!

As part of checking the scene, look to see if there are other victims. More help may be needed for multiple victims. Look also for any clues that may help you determine what happened and what first aid may be needed. As well, look for bystanders who may be able to help give first aid or go to a telephone to call 911.

Decide to Help

When you see a victim and the scene is safe, you need to decide to help that victim. This is not always easy. You may be worried about not doing the right thing, but remember that you have first aid training. Once you call for help, professionals will be there very soon. Your goal is to help the victim until they take over. Do not delay giving first aid because you hope someone else will do it—realize that it is up to you.

Call 911

Call 911 (or your local or company emergency number) immediately if you recognize a life-threatening injury or illness. A life-threatening emergency is one in which a problem threatens the victim's airway, breathing, or circulation of blood, as described later in this chapter. Do not try to transport a victim to the emergency room yourself in such cases. Movement may worsen the victim's condition, or the victim may suddenly need additional care on the way. If you are not sure whether a situation is serious enough to call, do not hesitate—call 911. It is better to be safe than sorry.

If the victim is responsive and may not be seriously injured or ill, go on to the next step to check the victim before calling 911—and then call 911 or a healthcare provider if needed.

Always call 911 when:

- The victim may have a life-threatening condition
- The victim is unresponsive
- The victim's condition may become life threatening
- Moving the victim could make the condition worse

Later chapters on first aid describe when to call 911 for other specific problems.

Remember that a victim may say his or her condition is not all that serious. For example, heart attack victims often say they just have "indigestion" even when they have other heart attack signs and symptoms. You should call 911 anyway and let the dispatch center decide when the situation is an emergency.

In addition to calling 911 for injury or illness, call in these situations:

- Fire, explosion
- Vehicle crash
- Downed electrical wire
- Chemical spill, gas leak, or the presence of any unknown substances

How to Call EMS

When you call 911 or your local emergency number, be ready to give the following information:

- Your name and the phone number you are using
- The location and number of victims—specific enough for the arriving crew to find them
- What happened to the victims and any special circumstances or conditions that may require special rescue or medical equipment
- The victim's condition: For example, is the victim responsive? Breathing? Bleeding?
- The victim's approximate age and sex
- What is being done for the victim(s)

It is important to not hang up until the dispatcher instructs you to, as you may be given advice on how to care for the victim.

If another responsible person is present, ask him or her to call 911 while you go on to check the victim and give first aid (**Figure 2-1**).

Check the Victim

Check the victim for life-threatening conditions requiring immediate first aid (see later section "Check the ABCs").

Give First Aid

Give first aid once you have checked the victim and know his or her condition. Later chapters give the first aid steps for the conditions you are likely to find. In most cases first aid involves simple actions you can take to help the victim. Note that first aiders do not give medications, even aspirin, to victims because of the risks of allergy or other complications. First aiders can, however, allow adult victims to take medications when appropriate, and in some cases first aiders may assist victims in taking their medications if needed.

Seek Medical Attention

You may have decided at first that the victim's condition was not an emergency and did not call 911. In many cases, however, the victim still needs to see a healthcare provider. If you have any doubt, call 911. Later chapters on specific conditions requiring first aid describe when a victim needs to go to the emergency room or see a healthcare provider.

Avoiding Infectious Disease

In any emergency situation there is some risk of a first aider getting an infectious disease from a victim who has a disease. That risk is very low, however, and taking steps to prevent being infected greatly reduces that risk.

Bloodborne Disease

Several serious diseases can be transmitted from one person to another through contact with the in-

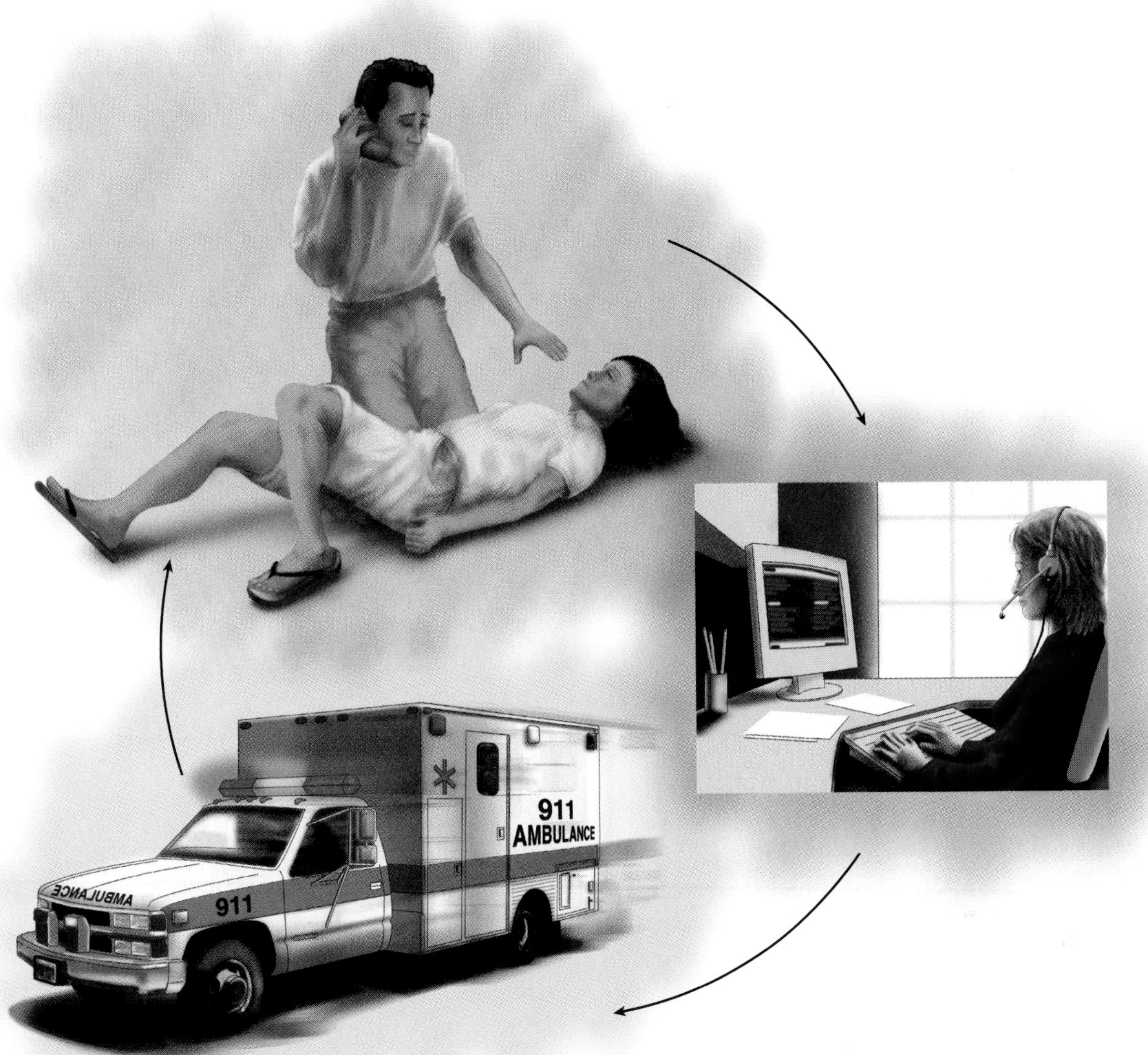

Figure 2-1 Call 911.

fected person's blood. These are called **bloodborne** diseases. Bacteria or viruses that cause such diseases, called **pathogens,** are also present in some other body fluids, such as semen, vaginal secretions, and bloody saliva or vomit. Other body fluids, such as nasal secretions, sweat, tears, and urine, do not normally transmit pathogens. Three serious bloodborne diseases are HIV, hepatitis B, and hepatitis C.

HIV

The human immunodeficiency virus (HIV) is the pathogen that eventually causes AIDS (acquired immunodeficiency syndrome). AIDS is a fatal disease transmitted from one person to another only through body fluids.

Hepatitis B

Hepatitis B (HBV) is a viral infectious disease of the liver also transmitted through contact with an infected person's body fluids. The disease is difficult to treat and often remains in the person for life, possibly leading to liver damage or cancer.

Learning Checkpoint 1

1. True or False: If you see victims injured in an emergency, the first thing to do is get to them quickly and check their condition.

2. When you encounter an injured victim, you should:

a. Give first aid until help arrives

b. Help a victim only if the scene is safe

c. Call 911 for life-threatening injuries

d. All of the above

3. Call 911 for:

a. Medical problems only

b. Police and fire services only

c. Medical problems and fires only

d. Medical problems and all emergencies

A vaccine is available for HBV. Individuals who are more likely to come in contact with HBV-infected people, such as healthcare workers and professional rescuers, often get this vaccine. The law requires that employees who are at risk for HBV be offered free vaccinations by their employer.

Hepatitis C

Hepatitis C (HCV) is another viral disease that can cause liver disease or cancer. It cannot be cured, and there is no vaccine.

Protection Against Bloodborne Disease

Because these bloodborne diseases cannot be cured, they should be prevented. The best prevention is to avoid contact with *all* victims' blood and body fluids. You cannot know whether a victim (even a close friend) is infected as often these diseases do not produce signs and symptoms. Even victims may not know that they are infected.

The Centers for Disease Control and Prevention (CDC) therefore recommends taking **universal precautions** whenever giving first aid. *Universal* means for all victims, all the time, and always assuming that blood and other body fluids may be infected. Use the following recommended precautions to prevent coming into contact with a victim's blood or body fluids:

- Use personal protective equipment
- If you do not have medical exam gloves with you, put your hands in plastic bags or

WEST NILE VIRUS

West Nile Virus (WNV) is a relatively new bloodborne disease now established as a seasonal epidemic in parts of North America. Less than 1% of people infected with WNV develop severe illness, however, and about 80% have no signs and symptoms at all. WNV is spread mostly by the bite of infected mosquitoes. The best way to avoid WNV is to prevent mosquito bites with personal protection such as wearing long sleeves and pants and reducing mosquito breeding sites.

have the victim dress his or her own wound

- Wash your hands with soap and water before and after giving first aid
- Keep a barrier (gloves or dry cloth) between body fluids and yourself
- Cover any cuts or scrapes in your skin with protective clothing or gloves
- Do not touch your mouth, nose, or eyes when giving first aid (e.g., do not eat, drink, or smoke)
- Do not touch objects soiled with blood or body fluids
- Be careful to avoid being cut by anything sharp at the emergency scene, such as broken glass or torn metal
- Use absorbent material to soak up spilled blood or body fluids, and dispose of it appropriately. Clean the area with a commercial disinfectant or a freshly made 10% bleach solution.
- If you are exposed to a victim's blood or body fluid, wash immediately with soap and water and call your healthcare provider. At work, report the situation to your supervisor.

OSHA requires use of universal precautions by employees who give first aid as part of their job.

Personal Protective Equipment

Personal protective equipment (PPE) is any equipment used to protect yourself from contact with blood or other body fluids. Most important, keep **medical exam gloves** in your first aid kit and wear them in most first aid situations (**Figure 2-2**).

A barrier device such as a pocket face mask or face shield is used when giving rescue breathing or cardiopulmonary resuscitation (CPR). This device should be in the first aid kit and should be used for added protection (**Figure 2-3**).

Other PPE devices include **eye protection, masks,** and **gowns or aprons**. These are not required in most first aid situations, although OSHA requires such protections be available in some workplaces. In such cases OSHA requires employees to be trained in the use of this PPE. Healthcare workers, for example, are required to wear masks and protective eyewear or face shields during procedures likely to generate droplets of blood or body fluids, and gowns or aprons when blood or body fluid may be splashed. These are called **standard precautions.**

Latex Gloves

Medical exam gloves are often made of latex rubber, to which some people are allergic. Signs and symptoms of latex allergy may include skin rashes, hives, itching eyes or skin, flushing, watery or swollen eyes, runny nose, or an asthmatic reaction. Use gloves made of vinyl or other material if you have any of these symptoms.

Airborne Disease

Infectious diseases may also be transmitted through the air, especially from a victim who

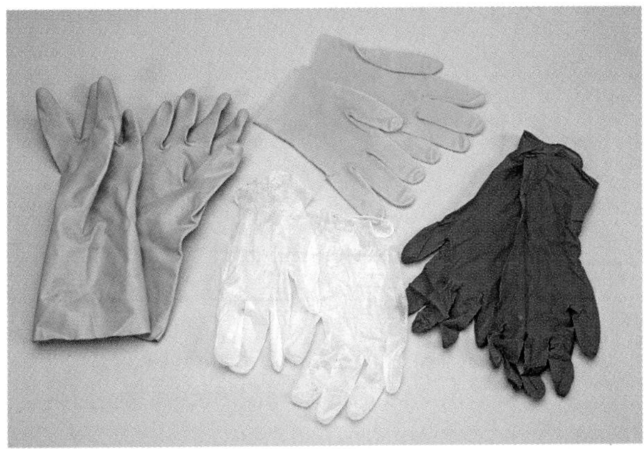

Figure 2-2 Wear gloves to protect yourself from contact with blood or other body fluids.

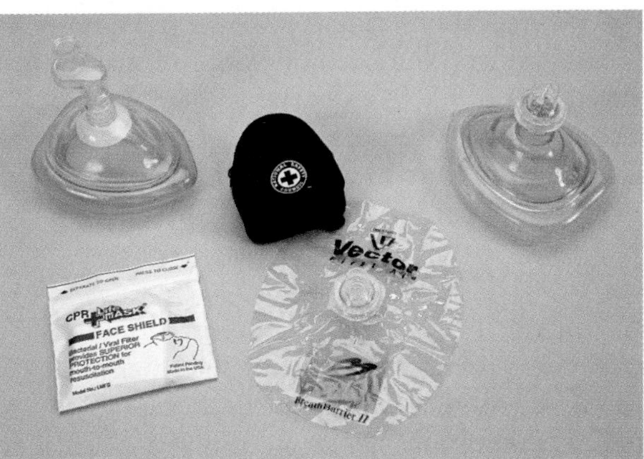

Figure 2-3 Variety of barrier devices.

Learning Checkpoint 2

1. True or False: Bloodborne diseases are transmitted only through contact with an infected person's blood.
2. True or False: The risk of getting a serious infectious disease by giving first aid is greatly reduced when you take precautions.
3. "Universal precautions" means:
   - **a.** Treat all victims as if their body fluids were infected
   - **b.** Always wear gloves if blood may be present
   - **c.** Do not touch your mouth, nose, or eyes when giving first aid
   - **d.** All of the above
4. Check off which of the following situations could lead to getting an infectious disease:
   - _____ **a.** Touching a bloody bandage in a trash can
   - _____ **b.** Shaking hands with a person with HIV
   - _____ **c.** Receiving a hepatitis B vaccination
   - _____ **d.** Not wearing gloves and giving first aid if you have a cut on your finger
   - _____ **e.** Being near a person with hepatitis C who is coughing
   - _____ **f.** Contact with an unresponsive victim

is coughing or sneezing. Tuberculosis (TB) has made a comeback in recent decades and is sometimes resistant to treatment.

Healthcare workers sometimes use precautions when caring for people known or suspected to have TB, but rarely does a first aider need to take special precautions against airborne disease.

First aiders who need or want to learn more about preventing bloodborne and airborne disease are encouraged to take the National Safety Council course on Bloodborne and Airborne Pathogens (www.nsc.org).

Check the Victim

As described earlier, after you recognize the emergency, check the scene for safety, and call 911 if appropriate, you then check the victim to see what problems may need first aid. This check, called an **assessment,** has three steps:

SARS

In 2003 an outbreak of severe acute respiratory syndrome (SARS) in some parts of the world caused a new scare. SARS is primarily an airborne infectious disease, transmitted when an infected person coughs or sneezes within close proximity of others. During the 2003 epidemic almost 10% of the approximately 8000 known SARS victims in the world died. Only 7 people in the U.S. were known to have contracted SARS, however, all during international travel to epidemic areas. The CDC continues to monitor the risks of SARS and will issue updates and warnings if new outbreaks occur.

1. Check for immediate life-threatening conditions (check the ABCs).
2. Get the victim's history (find out what happened and what may have contributed to the emergency).
3. Check the rest of the victim's body (perform a physical examination).

While giving first aid and waiting for help to arrive, continue with a fourth step:

4. Monitor the victim for any changes.

Always perform these steps in this order. If there is an immediate life-threatening problem, such as stopped breathing, the victim needs immediate help. This victim could die if you first spent time looking for broken bones or asking bystanders what happened. ***Always remember:*** Check the ABCs first!

Check the ABCs

In less than a minute you can check the victim for immediate life-threatening conditions. This is called "checking the ABCs," where:

A = Airway
B = Breathing
C = Circulation

We need these three things functioning to stay alive.

Begin your check of the ABCs by speaking to the victim as you approach. **A victim who can speak or cough has an open airway, is breathing, and has a beating heart.**

Unless the victim is obviously alert, **check for responsiveness.** Tap the victim on the shoulder and ask if he or she is okay. A victim is responsive if he or she can speak to you, move purposefully, or otherwise respond to stimuli. A victim who does not respond is called unresponsive. An unresponsive victim is considered to have a potentially life-threatening condition. If the victim is unresponsive, continue checking the ABCs.

A = Airway

We can breathe only if our airway is open. The airway may be blocked by something stuck in the throat or by an unresponsive victim's own tongue. To make sure the tongue is not obstructing the airway in an unresponsive victim, position the victim's head to open the airway. In a victim not suspected of having a neck injury, lift the chin and tilt the head back as shown in Figure 2-4. This is called the head tilt-chin lift.

If the victim may have a neck or spine injury (see Chapter 6), do not tilt the head back to open the airway. Instead, only lift the jaw upward using both hands (Figure 2-5). This is called a jaw thrust.

B = Breathing

After opening the airway you then check to see if the victim is breathing. Lean over with your ear close to the person's mouth and **look** at the victim's chest to see if it rises and falls with breathing. **Listen** for any sounds of breathing and **feel** for breath on your cheek. If you do not notice any signs of breathing within 10 seconds, assume the person is not breathing.

If you are trained in rescue breathing and cardiopulmonary resuscitation (CPR), at this point

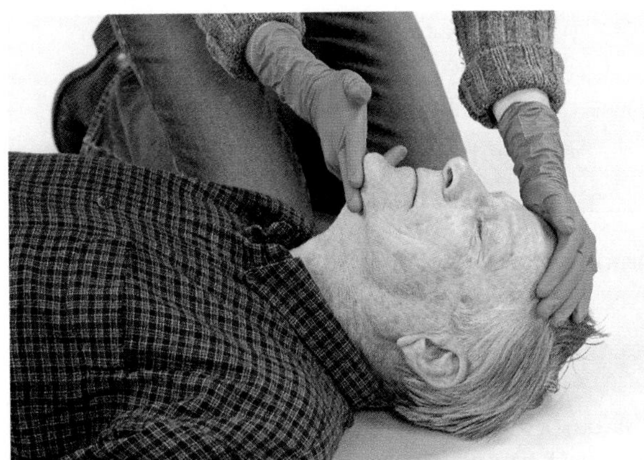

Figure 2-4 Head tilt-chin lift.

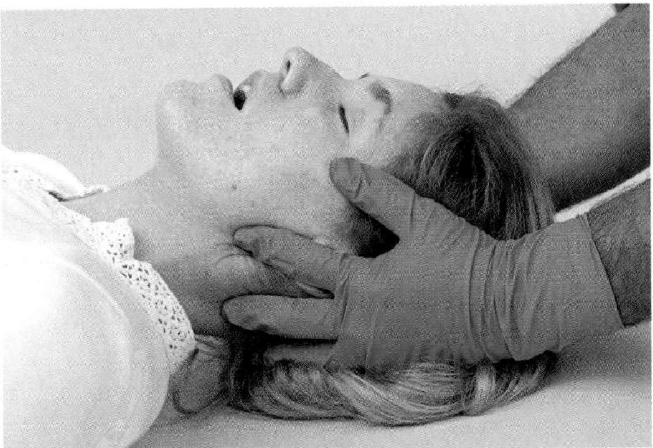

Figure 2-5 Jaw thrust.

you would give two slow breaths to a victim who is not breathing.

C = Circulation

After checking the victim's airway and breathing, you next check for circulation. This means checking that the heart is beating and blood is moving around the body (circulating). If the victim's heart has stopped or the victim is bleeding profusely, there is a circulation problem and the victim can die. **If the victim is moving, coughing, speaking, or breathing, the heart is beating.**

Check for signs of circulation by scanning the body for any signs of breathing, coughing, movement, and normal skin condition. Lack of circulation may be indicated by bluish, pale skin color, cool skin temperature, and clammy skin. It is currently recommended that *only healthcare workers or professional rescuers spend time checking for a victim's pulse.* Check for severe bleeding by quickly looking over the victim's body for obvious blood. Control any severe bleeding with direct pressure (see Chapter 3).

If you see no signs of circulation and you have been trained in CPR and the use of an AED, start CPR and call for an AED to be brought to the scene.

For more information see Appendix A. The National Safety Council course in CPR and AED is recommended. This course teaches what is called basic life support (BLS) techniques, including rescue breathing, CPR, choking care, and use of an automated electronic defibrillator (AED) for victims whose heart has stopped.

Get the Victim's History

After checking the ABCs for immediate life-threatening conditions, try to find out more about what happened and the victim's condition. Talk to a responsive victim, or ask bystanders about what they know or saw in a situation involving an unresponsive victim. Use the **SAMPLE** history format:

S = ***Signs and symptoms.*** What can you observe about the victim (**signs**)? Ask the victim how he or she feels (**symptoms**).

A = ***Allergies.*** Ask the victim about any allergies to foods, medicines, insect stings, or other substances. Look for a medical alert bracelet.

M = ***Medications.*** Ask the victim if he or she is taking any prescribed medications or over-the-counter products.

P = ***Previous problems.*** Ask the victim if he or she has had anything like this before or has any other illnesses.

L = ***Last food or drink.*** Ask the victim what and when he or she last ate or drank anything.

E = ***Events.*** Ask the victim what happened and try to identify the events that led to the current situation.

The information from a SAMPLE history may help you give the right first aid. If the victim is unresponsive when help arrives, give any information gathered to the EMS professionals. It will help them to give the appropriate medical care.

Physical Examination

The third step of the assessment of an injured or ill victim is the physical examination. With this examination you may find other injuries that need first aid or additional clues to a victim's condition. It is important to note, however, that you do not stop giving first aid for a serious condition just to do or complete this examination. Instead, keep the victim still and calm and wait for EMS professionals to examine the victim.

The physical examination includes examining the victim from head to toe looking for anything out of the ordinary. As a general rule look for the following signs and symptoms of injury or illness throughout the body:

- Pain when an area is touched
- Bleeding or other wounds
- An area that is swollen or deformed from usual appearance
- Skin color (flushed or pale), temperature (hot or cold), moisture (dry, sweating, clammy)
- Abnormal sensation or movement of the area

Monitor the Victim

Give first aid for injuries or illness you discover in your assessment. With very minor conditions the victim may need no more than your first

Perform the Skill

Check the ABCs

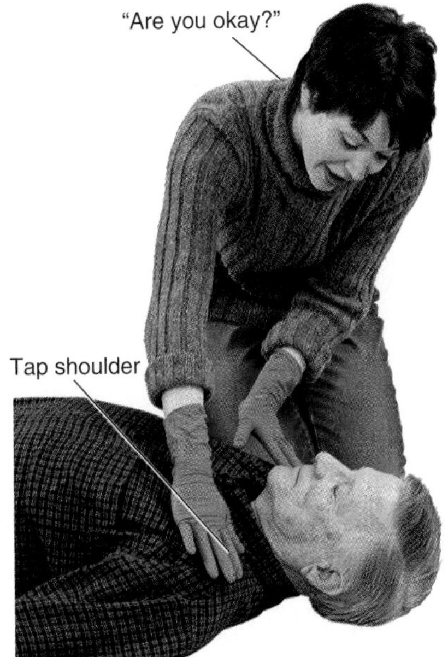
"Are you okay?"
Tap shoulder

1 Check responsiveness.

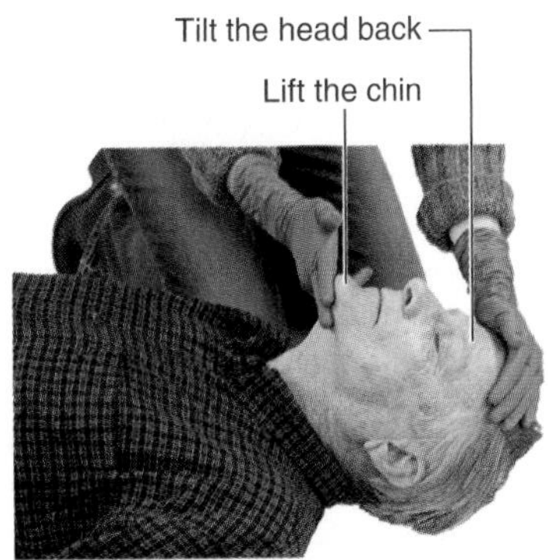
Tilt the head back
Lift the chin

2 Open the airway.

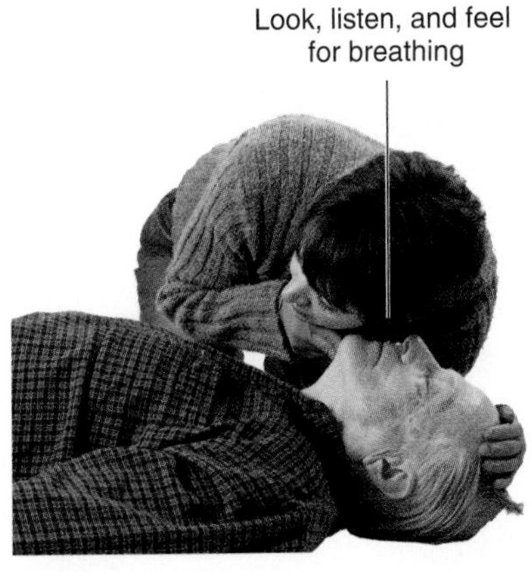
Look, listen, and feel for breathing

3 Check for breathing.

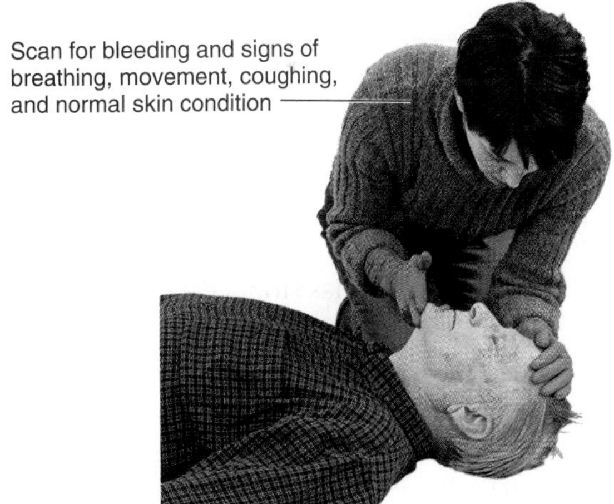
Scan for bleeding and signs of breathing, movement, coughing, and normal skin condition

4 Check for signs of circulation.

aid. In other situations the victim may need to see a healthcare provider or go to an emergency room. With all life-threatening or serious conditions, you should have called 911 and will now be awaiting the arrival of help.

While waiting, monitor the victim to make sure the condition does not worsen. With an unresponsive victim or a victim with a serious injury, repeat your assessment of the ABCs at least every 5 minutes.

Perform the Skill

Physical Examination of Injured Victim

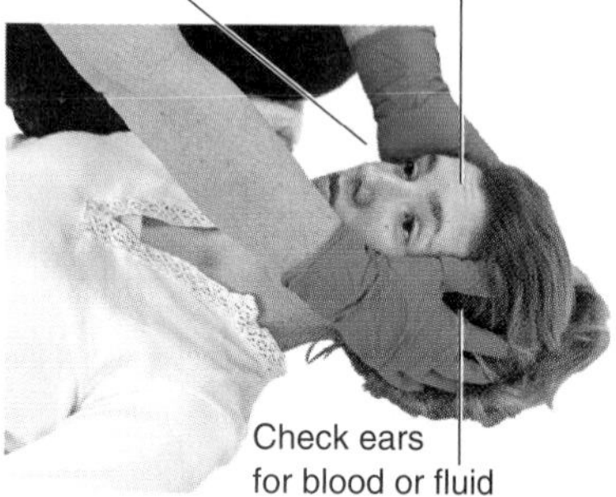
Check pupils: equal size, react to light
Check for bleeding, swelling, or depressed area
Check ears for blood or fluid

1 Being careful not to move the victim's head or neck, check the head.

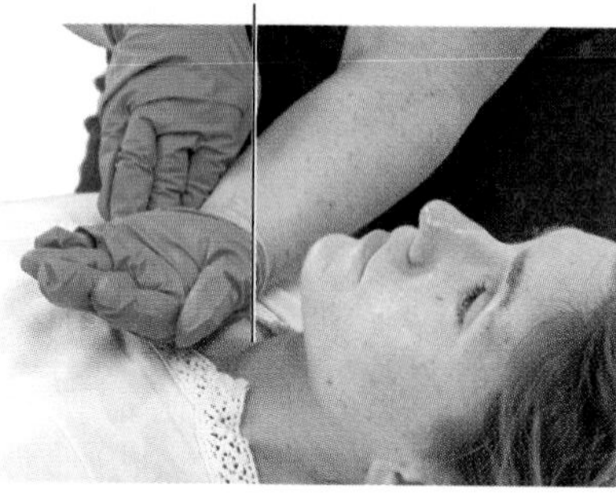
Do not move the neck

2 Check neck area for medical alert necklace, deformity or swelling, and pain. *Do not move the neck.*

Check skin for color, temperature, and moisture

3 Check skin appearance, temperature, moisture.

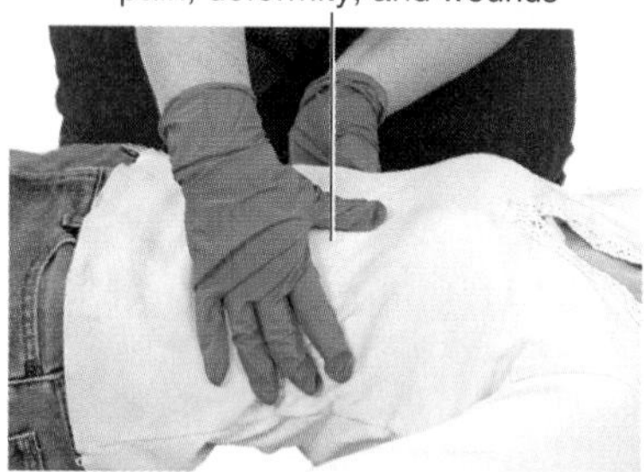
Check for movement with breathing, pain, deformity, and wounds

4 Check chest. Ask victim to breathe deeply.

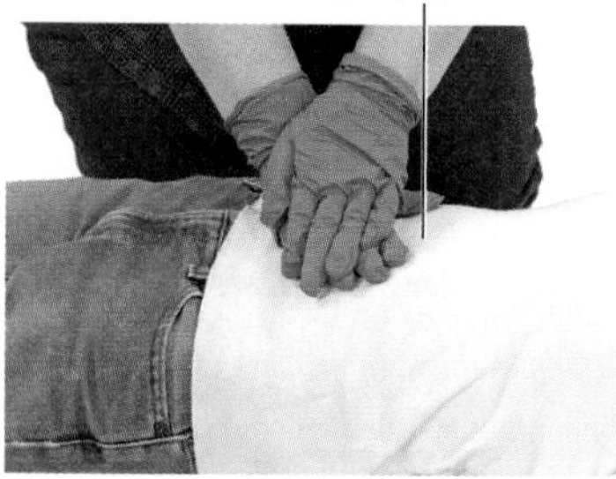
Gently check for rigidity, pain, or bleeding

5 Check abdomen.

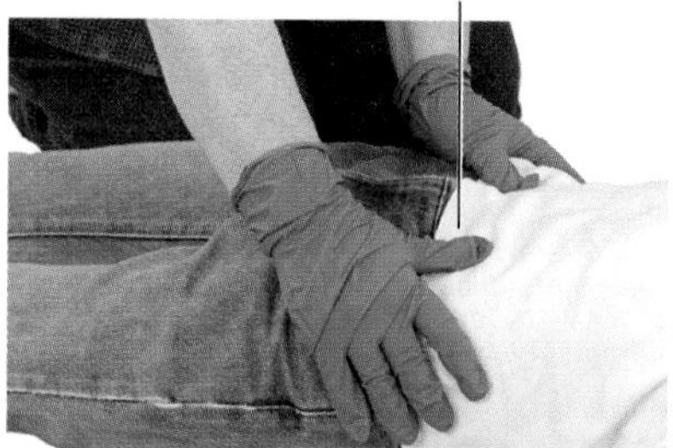
Gently squeeze pelvis to detect pain or deformity

6 Check pelvis and hips.

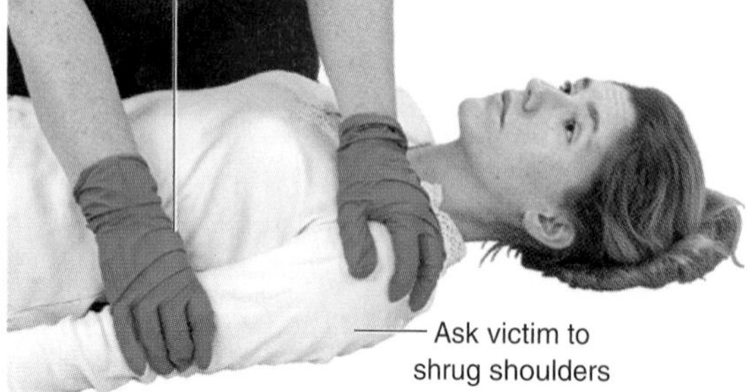
Ask victim to move arm, check from shoulder to fingers for sensation, pain, deformity, and bleeding
Ask victim to shrug shoulders

7 Check upper extremities. Look for medical alert bracelet.

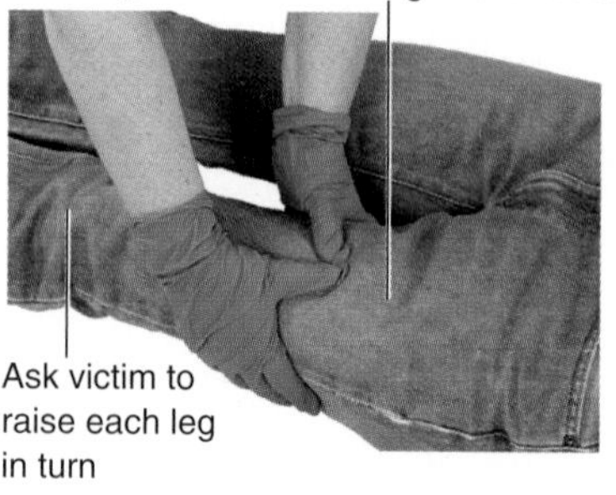
Feel each leg from thigh to toes for sensation, pain, deformity, and bleeding. Check feet for signs of circulation problems (cold, blue).
Ask victim to raise each leg in turn

8 Check lower extremities.

Learning Checkpoint 3

1. You first encounter a victim lying quietly on the floor. Number the following actions in the correct order.

_____ **a.** Check victim for signs of circulation

_____ **b.** Listen near victim's mouth for breathing sounds

_____ **c.** Check to see if victim responds to your voice or touch

_____ **d.** Position the victim to open the airway

2. Describe three ways you can detect if a victim is breathing.

____

3. True or False: If you hear a victim coughing or breathing, you can assume the heart is beating.

4. Write what each letter in the SAMPLE history stands for:

S = ____________

A = ____________

M = ____________

P = ____________

L = ____________

E = ____________

5. Describe what signs and symptoms of injury you are looking for as you examine each part of a victim's body.

____

6. As you do a physical examination of an unresponsive victim, what one body area should you be very careful not to move?

____

The Recovery Position

An unresponsive victim who is breathing when found or after you open the airway should be put in the recovery position while waiting for help to arrive (**Figure 2-6**). This position:

- Helps keep the airway open
- Allows fluids to drain from the mouth
- Prevents inhaling stomach contents if the victim vomits

Once in the recovery position, continue to monitor the victim's breathing.

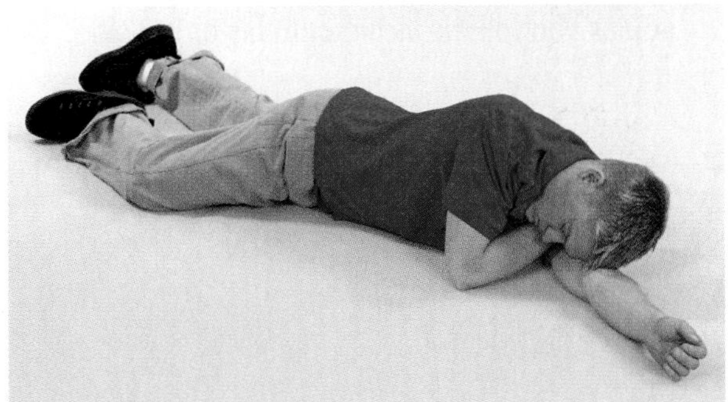

Figure 2-6 The recovery position.

Perform the Skill

Recovery Position

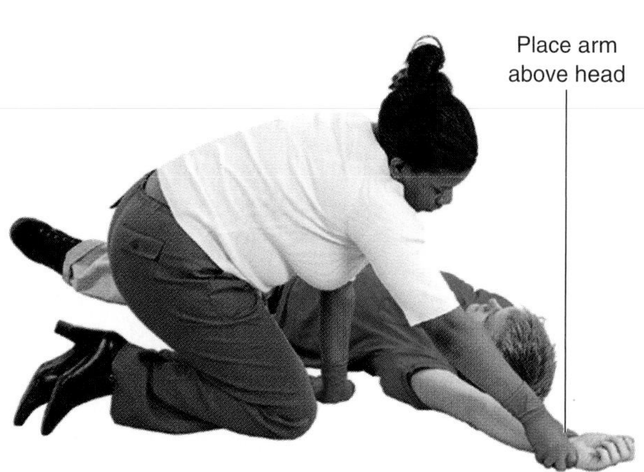

Place arm
above head

1 Position the victim's arm.

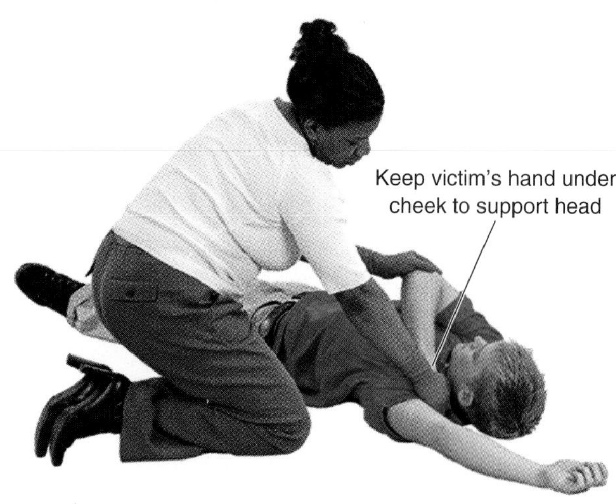

Keep victim's hand under
cheek to support head

2 Move victim's other arm across chest and against cheek.

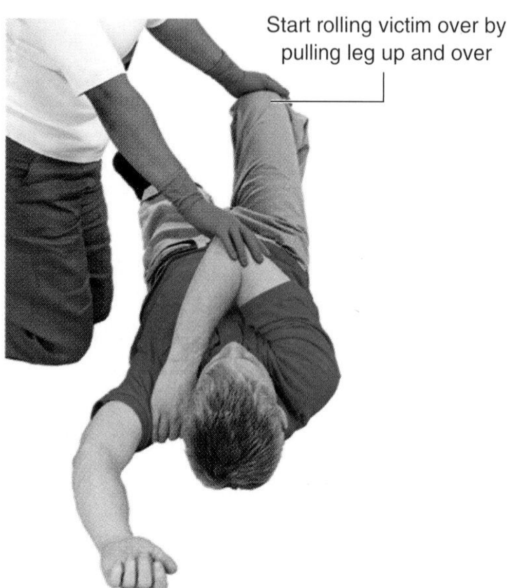
Start rolling victim over by
pulling leg up and over

3 Bend the victim's leg at the knee and pull it toward you as you roll the victim onto his or her side.

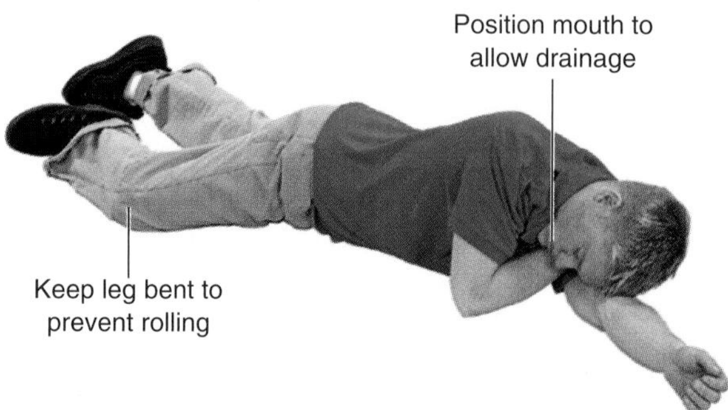

Position mouth to
allow drainage
Keep leg bent to
prevent rolling

4 Adjust victim's position as needed.

Chapter

3 Bleeding and Wound Care

CHAPTER PREVIEW

- Controlling External Bleeding
- Wound Care
- Dressings
- Bandages
- Internal Bleeding

Many injuries cause external or internal bleeding. Bleeding may be minor or life threatening. In addition to controlling bleeding, first aiders should know how to care for different kinds of wounds and how to apply dressings and bandages.

Types of External Bleeding

There are three types of external bleeding (**Figure 3-1**):

- **Bleeding from injured arteries** is generally more serious and is more likely with deep injuries. The blood is bright red and may spurt from the wound and blood loss can be very rapid. This bleeding needs to be controlled immediately.
- **Bleeding from injured veins** is generally slower and steady but can still be serious. The blood is dark red and flows steadily rather than spurting. This bleeding is usually easier to control.
- **Bleeding from capillaries** occurs with shallow cuts or scrapes and often stops soon by itself. The wound still needs attention to prevent infection.

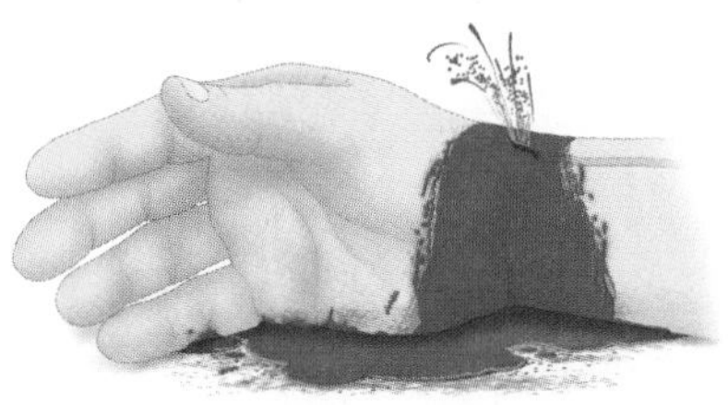

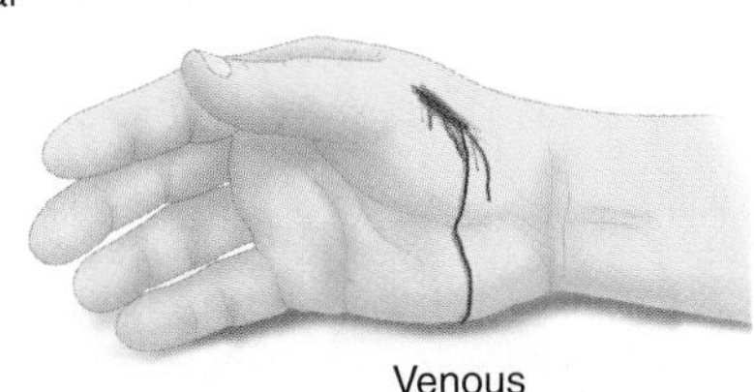

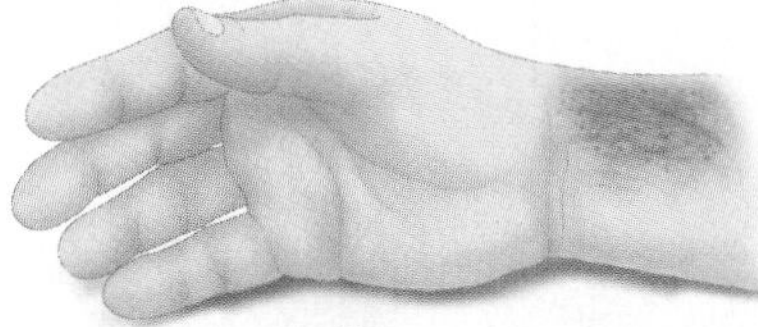

Figure 3-1 Arterial, venous, and capillary bleeding.

Controlling External Bleeding

For minor bleeding, clean and dress the wound (as described later). Usually the bleeding stops by itself or with light pressure on the dressing. For more serious bleeding, give first aid *immediately* to stop the bleeding.

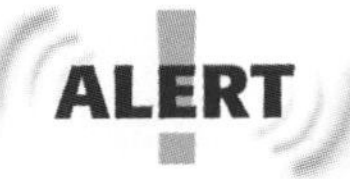

Bleeding

Use your bare hands only if no barrier is available, and then wash immediately.
Do not put pressure on an object in a wound.
Do not put pressure on the scalp if the skull may be injured.
Do not use a tourniquet to stop bleeding except as an extreme last resort (limb will likely be lost).

Perform the Skill

Controlling Bleeding

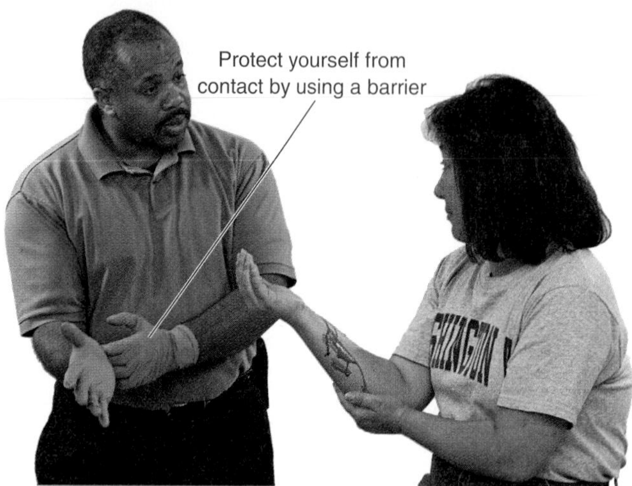
Protect yourself from contact by using a barrier

1 Put on gloves.

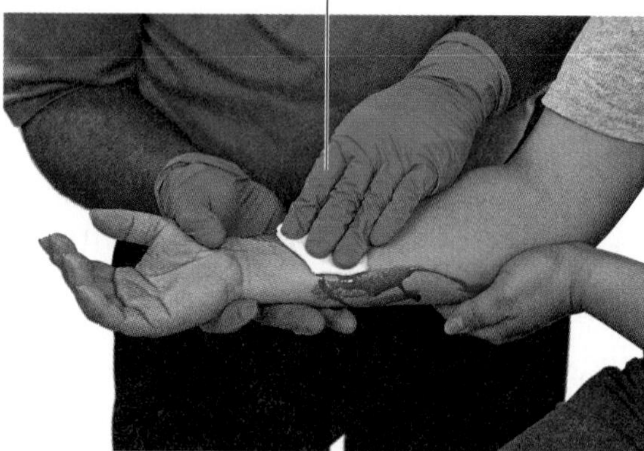
Apply pressure directly on wound

2 Place a sterile dressing on the wound and apply direct pressure with your hand.

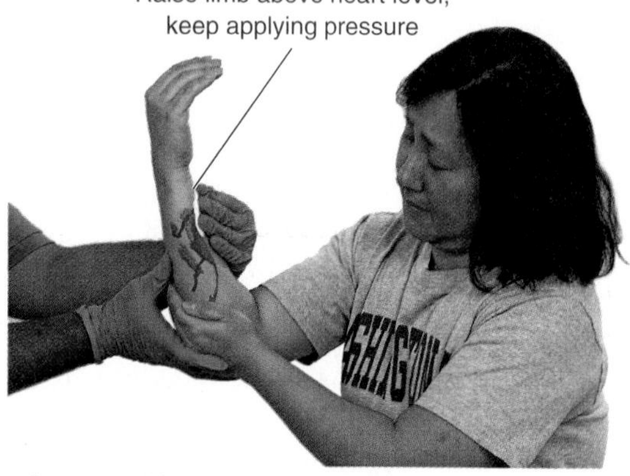
Raise limb above heart level; keep applying pressure

3 Elevate a bleeding arm or leg to help slow the bleeding.

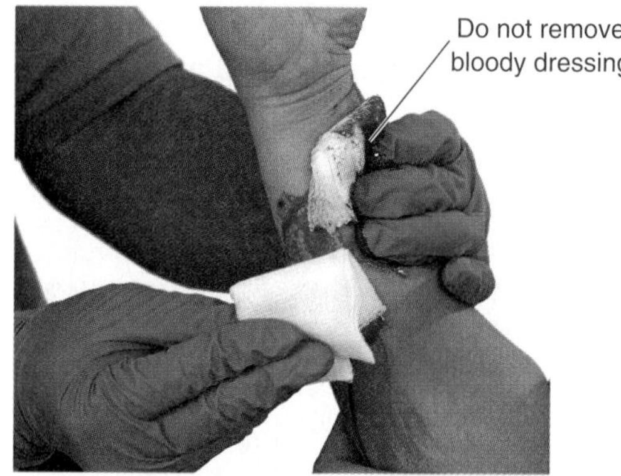
Do not remove bloody dressing

4 If needed, put another dressing or cloth pad on top of the first and keep applying pressure.

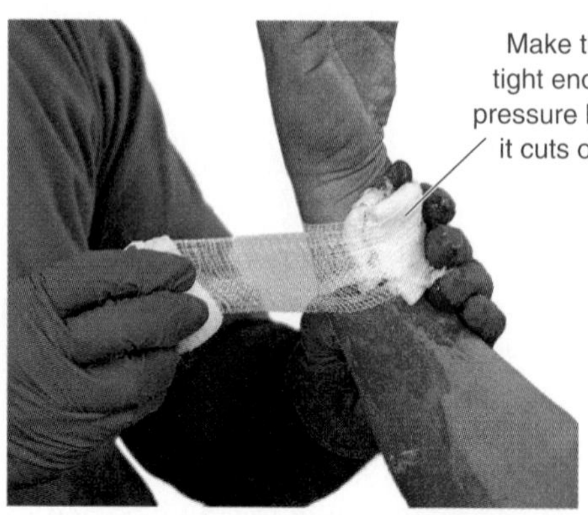
Make the bandage tight enough to apply pressure but not so tight it cuts off circulation

5 Apply a roller bandage to keep pressure on the wound.

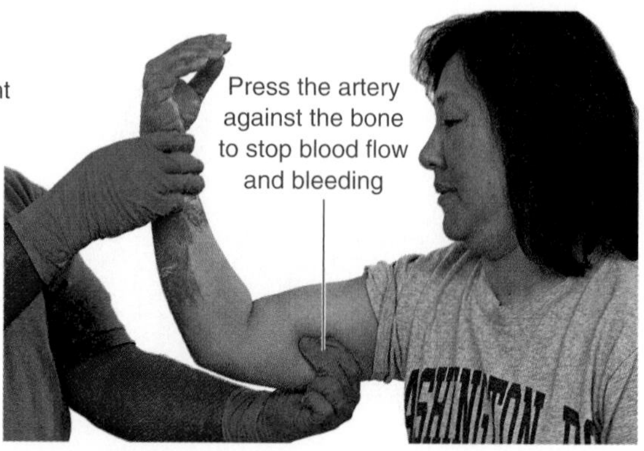
Press the artery against the bone to stop blood flow and bleeding

6 If needed, apply pressure at pressure point.

When You See

- Bleeding from a wound
- Blood on a victim
- Shock: pale, clammy skin

Do This First

1. Put on medical exam gloves or use another barrier to protect yourself from contact with the blood (such as dressings, a plastic bag, or the victim's own hand).
2. Move aside any clothing and place a sterile dressing (or clean cloth) on the wound, then apply direct pressure on the wound with your hand.
3. With a bleeding arm or leg, raise the limb above the heart level while keeping pressure on the wound. Be careful moving the victim because of the possibility of other injuries.
4. If blood soaks through the dressing, do not remove the old dressing but put another dressing or cloth pad on top of it and keep applying pressure.
5. If possible, wrap a roller bandage around the limb to hold the dressings in place and apply pressure. Be careful not to cut off circulation to the limb.
6. If direct pressure does not control the bleeding, also apply indirect pressure at a pressure point in the arm or leg to squeeze the artery closed (Figure 3-2).

Additional Care

- Call 911
- Treat the victim for shock (see Chapter 4)
- Do not remove the dressings/bandage. The wound will be cleaned later by medical personnel.

Learning Checkpoint 1

1. True or False: Arterial bleeding is the most serious because blood loss can be very rapid.

2. True or False: The first thing to do with any bleeding wound is wash it and apply antibiotic ointment.

3. Number the steps for bleeding control in correct order:

_____ Use indirect pressure

_____ Put direct pressure on wound using a dressing

_____ Put on gloves

_____ Apply additional dressings

_____ Apply pressure bandage

_____ Elevate limb

4. Describe the skin characteristics of a victim who has been bleeding severely.

____

5. If you do not have medical exam gloves with you, what other materials or objects can be used as a barrier between your hand and the wound when applying direct pressure?

____

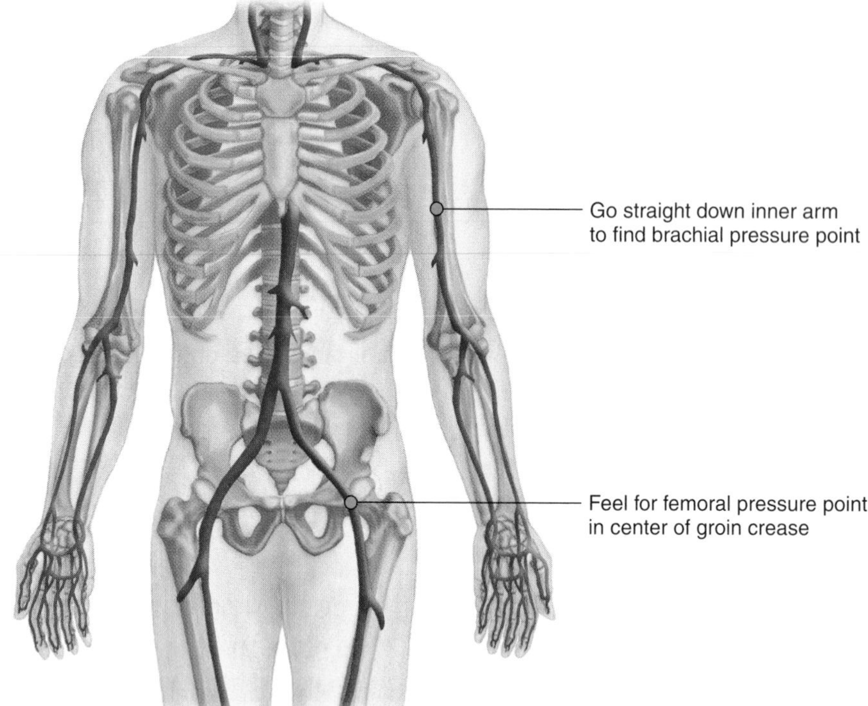
Go straight down inner arm
to find brachial pressure point
Feel for femoral pressure point
in center of groin crease

Figure 3-2 Use indirect pressure on pressure points to stop bleeding.

Wound Care

Wound care involves cleaning and dressing a wound to prevent infection and protect the wound so that healing can occur. Remember: *Do not waste time cleaning a wound that is severely bleeding. Controlling the bleeding is the priority.* Healthcare personnel will clean the wound as needed.

The main types of open wounds include the following:

- **Abrasions** occur when the top skin is scraped off. Foreign material may be present in the wound that can cause infection (**Figure 3-3**).
- **Lacerations**, or cuts, may be straight-edged (incision) or jagged, and may cause heavier bleeding (**Figure 3-4**).
- **Punctures** of the skin are caused by a sharp object penetrating down into the skin and possibly deeper tissues and are more likely to trap foreign material in the body (**Figure 3-5**).
- **Avulsions** are areas of skin or other tissue torn partially from the body, like a flap (**Figure 3-6**).

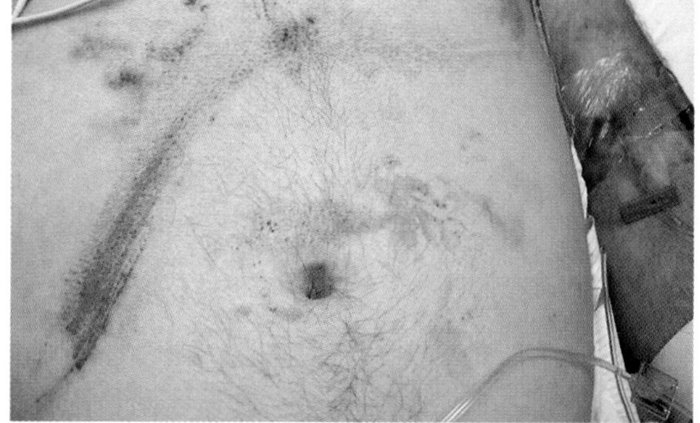

Figure 3-3 Abrasion.

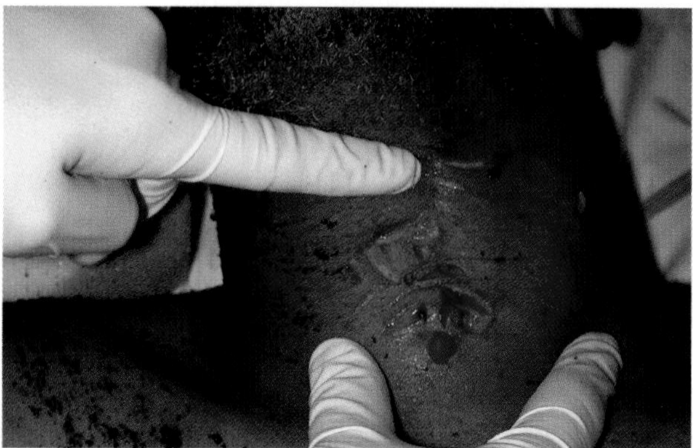

Figure 3-4 Laceration.

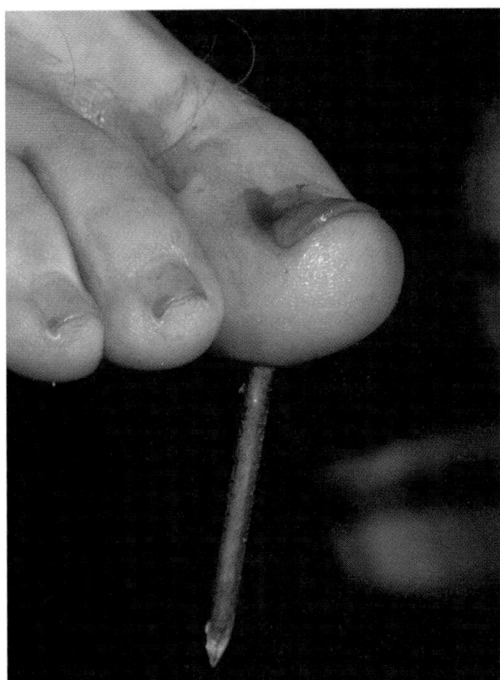

Figure 3-5 Puncture.

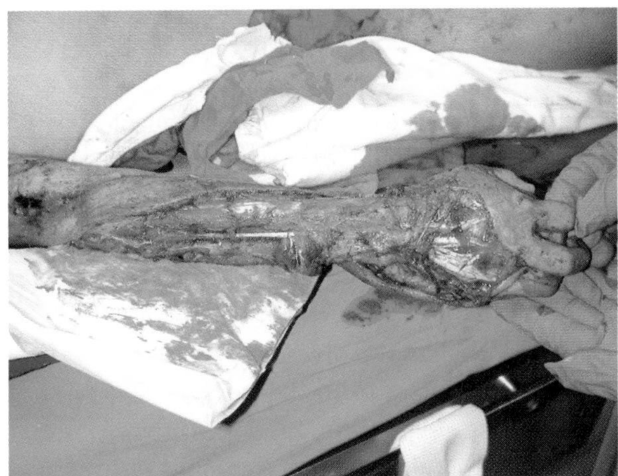

Figure 3-6 Avulsion.

Other special wounds are described in the following pages.

Cleaning Wounds

Unless the wound is very large or bleeding seriously, or the victim has other injuries needing attention, clean the wound to help prevent infection. Wash your hands first and wear gloves if available.

When You See

- An open wound

Do This First

1. Gently wash the wound with soap and water to remove dirt.
2. Use tweezers to remove any small particles.
3. Pat the area dry. With abrasions only, apply an antibiotic ointment.
4. Cover the wound with a sterile dressing and bandage (or adhesive bandage with nonstick pad).

Additional Care

- If stitches may be needed (see later section), or if the victim does not have a current tetanus vaccination, seek medical attention
- Change the dressing daily or if it becomes wet. (If a dressing sticks to the wound, soak it in water first.) Seek medical attention if the wound later looks infected.

Wound Infection

Any wound can become infected (Figure 3-7). The victim should then seek medical attention. The signs and symptoms of a wound infection are:

- Wound area is red, swollen, and warm
- Pain
- Pus
- Fever
- Red streaks or trails on the skin near the wound are a sign the infection is spreading—see a healthcare provider immediately

Wound Cleaning

Do not try to clean a major wound after controlling bleeding—it may start bleeding again.
Healthcare personnel will clean the wound as needed.
Do not use alcohol, hydrogen peroxide, or iodine on the wound.
Avoid breathing on the wound.

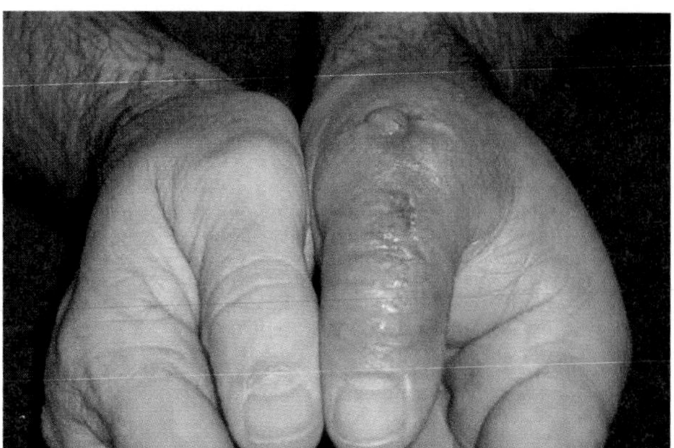

Figure 3-7 An infected wound.

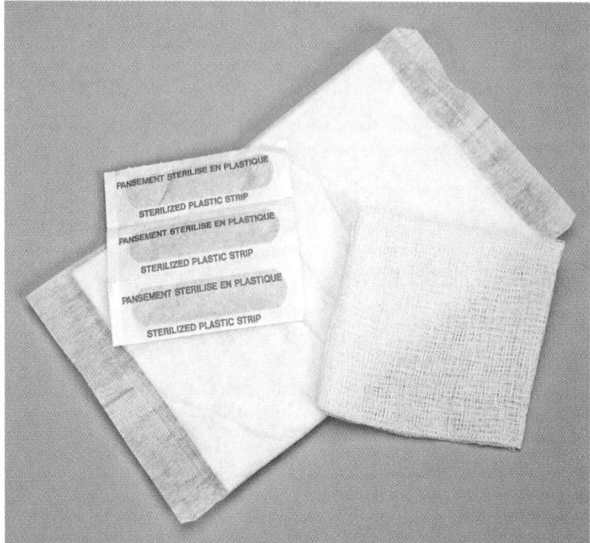

Figure 3-8 A variety of dressings.

With any deep or puncture wound, the risk of tetanus—a very serious infection—must be considered. Adults need a tetanus booster at least every 10 years, and a tetanus booster may be recommended before 10 years if there is an injury. Seek medical attention for any deep or puncture wound.

Dressing Wounds

Dressings are put on wounds to help stop bleeding, prevent infection, and protect the wound while healing. First aid kits should include sealed sterile gauze dressings in many sizes. Adhesive strips such as Band-Aids® are dressings combined with a

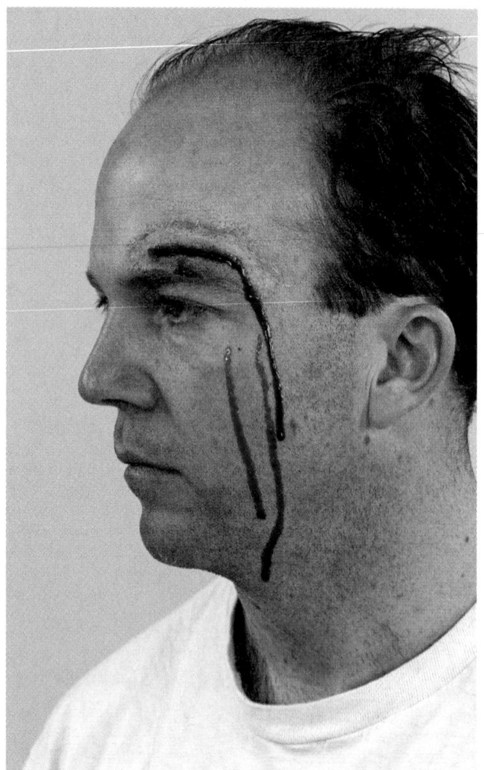

Figure 3-9 A large open wound that may require stitches.

bandage. If a sterile dressing is not available, use a clean, nonfluffy cloth as a dressing (**Figure 3-8**).

After washing and drying the wound, apply the dressing this way:

1. Wash hands and wear gloves.
2. Choose a dressing larger than the wound.
3. Carefully lay the dressing on the wound (do not slide it on from the side).
4. If blood seeps through, do not remove the dressing but add more dressings on top.
5. Apply a bandage to hold the dressing in place (see later section on bandaging).

When to Seek Medical Attention

Remember to call 911 for severe bleeding. In addition, see a healthcare provider as soon as possible for these wounds:

- Bleeding is not easily controlled
- Any deep or large wound
- Significant wounds on the face (**Figure 3-9**)
- Signs and symptoms that the wound is infected

- Any bite from an animal or human
- Foreign object or material embedded in the wound
- The victim is unsure about tetanus vaccination
- The victim may need stitches for:
  - Cuts on the face or hands when the edges do not close together
  - Gaping wounds
  - Cuts longer than 1 inch

Special Wounds

Puncture Wounds

Puncture wounds have a greater risk of infection because often they bleed less and therefore germs may not be flushed out. In addition to routine wound care, follow these steps:

1. Remove any small objects or dirt but not larger impaled objects (see next section).
2. Gently press on wound edges to promote bleeding.
3. Do not put any medication inside or over the puncture wound.
4. Wash the wound well in running water directed at the puncture site.
5. Dress the wound and seek medical attention.

Impaled Objects

Removing an object from a wound could cause more injury and bleeding. Leave it in place and dress the wound around it (**Figure 3-10**):

1. Control bleeding by applying direct pressure at the sides of the object.
2. Dress the wound around the object.
3. Pad the object in place with large dressings or folded cloths.
4. Support the object while bandaging it in place.
5. Seek medical attention.

Amputations

In an amputation injury a body part has been severed from the body. Control the bleeding and care for the victim's wound first, then recover and care for the amputated part. Follow these steps:

1. Wrap the severed part in a dry sterile dressing or clean cloth. Do not wash it.
2. Place the part in a plastic bag and seal it.
3. Place the sealed bag in another bag or container with ice. Do not let the part touch ice directly, and do not surround it with ice (**Figure 3-11**).
4. Make sure the severed part is given to the responding crew or taken with the victim to the emergency room.

Genital Injuries

Provide privacy for a victim with bleeding or injury in the genital area. Follow these guidelines:

- Use direct pressure to control external bleeding

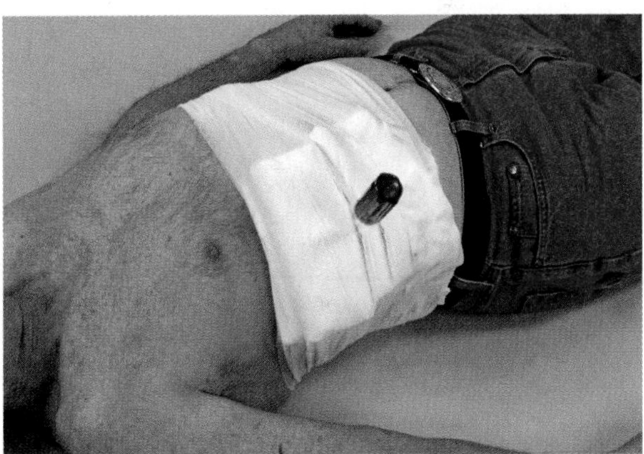

Figure 3-10 Leave an impaled object in place but keep it from moving.

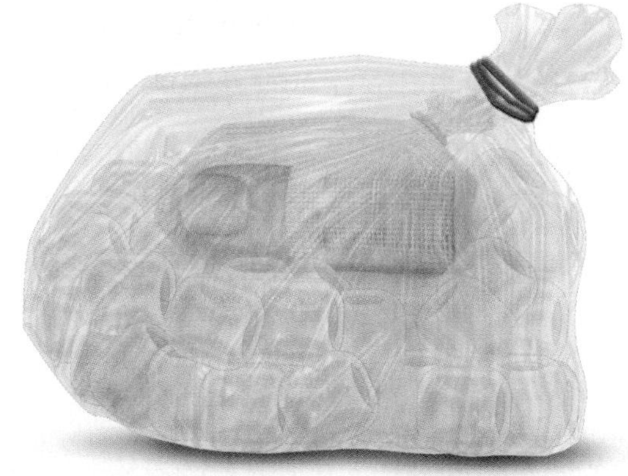

Figure 3-11 Keep amputated part cold but not directly touching ice.

Learning Checkpoint 2

1. Check off the actions below to include in wound care:

_____ Wash minor wounds with soap and water

_____ Pour rubbing alcohol on any wound

_____ Wash major wounds to help stop the bleeding

_____ Use tweezers to remove dirt particles from a minor wound

_____ Cover any wound with a sterile dressing and bandage

_____ Let a scab form before washing a minor wound

_____ See a healthcare provider for a deep or puncture wound

_____ Blow on a minor wound to cool the area and relieve pain

2. If you are changing a wound dressing a day after the injury and the dressing sticks to the wound, what should you do?

____

3. True or False: Puncture wounds have little risk for infection.

4. True or False: You don't need to bother putting on gloves to dress a minor wound if you know the victim well.

5. For what type of wound is an antibiotic ointment appropriate?

____

6. Check off which signs and symptoms may indicate a wound is infected:

_____ Headache

_____ Red, swollen area

_____ Cool, clammy skin

_____ Nausea and vomiting

_____ Warmth in the area

_____ Fever

_____ A scab forms that looks dark brown

_____ Pus drains from the wound

7. Which of these victims need to seek medical attention? (Check all that apply.)

_____ Jose has a deep laceration from a piece of equipment, but you managed to stop the bleeding in 15 minutes.

_____ Rebecca had lunch in a nearby park and was bitten by a squirrel she was feeding, but the bleeding stopped almost immediately.

_____ Carl scraped his knee when he fell off his bicycle on the way to work, but the abrasion washed out clean and you have applied an antibiotic ointment.

_____ Kim got a bad gash on her cheek when a bottle broke in the supply room, but she had already stopped the bleeding by the time you saw her.

- For injured testicles, provide support with a towel between the legs like a diaper
- For vaginal bleeding, have the woman press a sanitary pad or clean folded towel to the area
- Call 911 for severe or continuing bleeding, significant pain or swelling, or the possibility of sexual abuse

Head and Face Wounds

Injuries to the head or face may require special first aid. The following sections list guidelines for these special injuries.

With any significant injury to the head, the victim may also have a neck or spinal injury (see Chapter 6). If you suspect a spinal injury, be careful not to move the victim's head while giving first aid for head and face wounds.

Skull Injuries

If the victim is bleeding from the head, consider the additional possibility of a skull fracture if the victim had a blow to the head.

When You See

- A deformed area of the skull
- A depressed area in the bone felt during the physical examination
- Blood or fluid from the ears or nose
- Object impaled in the skull

Do This First

1. If the victim is unresponsive, check the ABCs.
2. *Do not clean the wound, press on it, or remove an impaled object.*
3. Cover the wound with a sterile dressing.
4. If there is significant bleeding, apply pressure only around the edges of the wound, not on the wound itself.
5. Do not move the victim unnecessarily, since there may also be a spinal injury.

Additional Care

- Call 911 and stay with the victim
- Put an unresponsive victim in the recovery position (unless there may be a spinal injury)
- Seek medical attention if the victim later experiences nausea and vomiting, persistent headache, drowsiness or disorientation, stumbling or lack of coordination, or problems with speech or vision

Head Wounds Without Suspected Skull Fracture

When You See

- Bleeding from the head
- No sign of skull fracture

Do This First

1. Replace any skin flaps and cover the wound with a sterile dressing.
2. Use direct pressure to control bleeding.
3. Put a roller or triangle bandage around the victim's head to secure the dressing (Figure 3-12).

Additional Care

- Position the victim with head and shoulders raised to help control bleeding

Eye Injuries

Eye injuries can be serious because vision may be affected.

For a blow to the eye:

1. If the eye is bleeding or leaking fluid, call 911 or get the victim to the emergency room immediately.
2. Put a cold pack over the eye for 15 minutes to ease pain and reduce swelling, but do not put pressure on the eye. If the victim is wearing a contact lens, do not remove it (Figure 3-13).
3. Have victim lie still and also cover the uninjured eye. Movement of the uninjured eye causes movement of the injured one.
4. Seek medical attention if pain persists or vision is affected in any way.

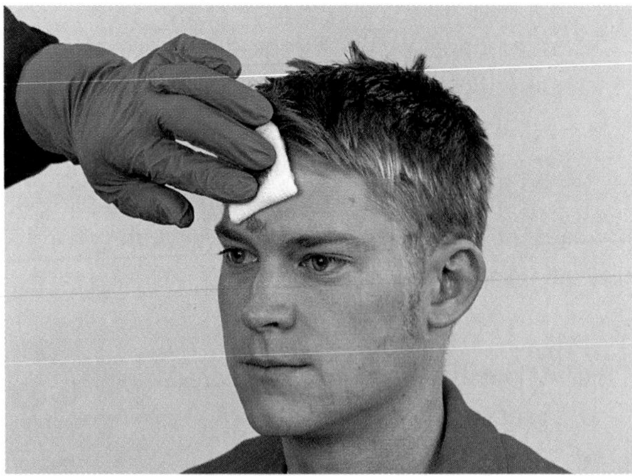

(a) Place dressing against wound.

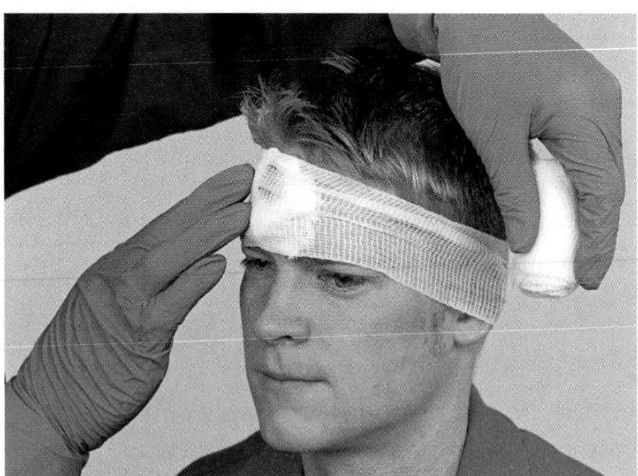

(b) A roller bandage secures the pressure dressing in place.

Figure 3-12 Dressing a head wound.

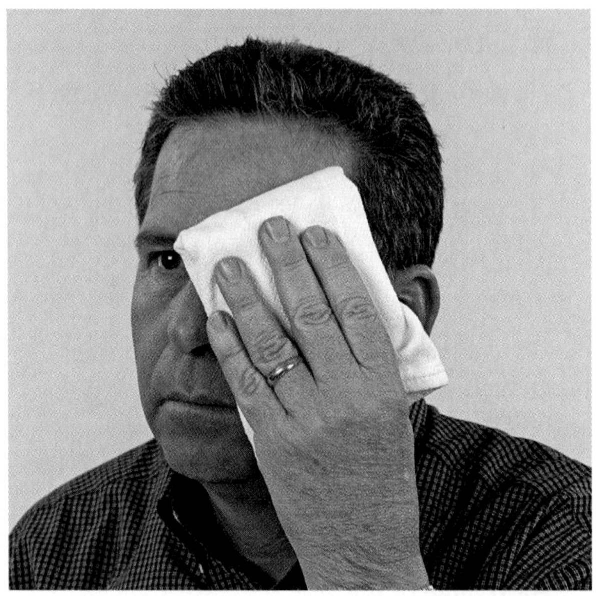

Figure 3-13 For a blow to the eye, hold a cold pack on the eye.

For an embedded object in the eye:

1. Do not remove the object. Stabilize it in place with dressings or bulky cloth.
2. Cover both eyes because movement of the uninjured one causes movement of the injured one.
3. Call 911 or get the victim to the emergency room immediately.

For dirt or a small particle in the eye:

1. Do not let victim rub the eye.

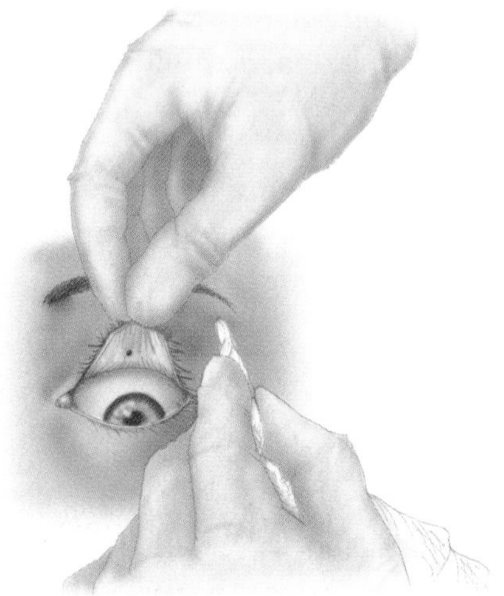

Figure 3-14 Carefully remove a particle from the eyelid.

2. Gently pull the upper eyelid out and down over the lower eyelid.
3. If the particle remains, gently flush the eye with water from a medicine dropper or water glass. Have the victim hold head with the affected eye lower than the other so that water does not flow into the unaffected eye.
4. If the particle remains and is visible, carefully try to brush it out with a sterile dressing. Lift the upper eyelid and swab its underside if you see the particle (**Figure 3-14**).
5. If the particle still remains or the victim has any vision problems or pain, cover the eye with a sterile dressing and seek medi-

cal attention. Also cover the uninjured eye, because movement of the uninjured eye causes movement of the injured one.

For a chemical or substance splashed in the eye:

1. Rinse the eye with running water for 20 minutes.
2. Have the victim hold head with the affected eye lower than the other so that water does not flow into the unaffected eye. (See Chapter 5 on chemical burns.)

Ear Injuries

With bleeding from the external ear, control the bleeding with direct pressure and dress the wound. For bleeding from within the ear, follow these guidelines:

When You See

- Bleeding inside the ear
- Signs of pain
- Possible deafness

Do This First

1. If the blood looks watery, this could mean a skull fracture. Call 911.
2. Help victim to sit up, tilting the affected ear lower to let blood drain out.
3. Cover the ear with a loose sterile dressing, but do not apply pressure.
4. Seek medical attention immediately.

Additional Care

- Keep the ear covered to reduce the risk of infection

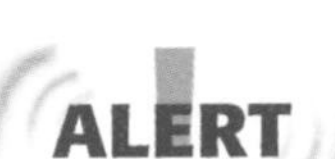

Ear Wound

Do not plug the ear closed to try to stop bleeding.

Nose Injuries

When You See

- Blood coming from either or both nostrils
- Blood possibly running from back of nose down into the mouth or throat

Do This First

1. Have victim sit and tilt head slightly forward with mouth open. Carefully remove any object you see in the nose.
2. Have victim pinch the nostrils together just below the bridge of the nose for 10 minutes (Figure 3-15). Ask victim to breathe through the mouth and not speak, swallow, cough, or sniff.
3. If victim is gasping or choking on blood in the throat, call 911.
4. After 10 minutes, release the pressure slowly. Pinch the nostrils again for another 10 minutes if bleeding continues.
5. Place a cold compress on the bridge of the nose.

Additional Care

- Seek medical attention if:
  - bleeding continues after two attempts to control bleeding
  - you suspect the nose is broken
  - the victim has high blood pressure
- Have the person rest for a few hours and avoid rubbing or blowing the nose

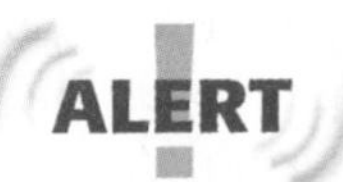

Nosebleed

Do not tilt the victim's head backward. Do not have the victim lie down.

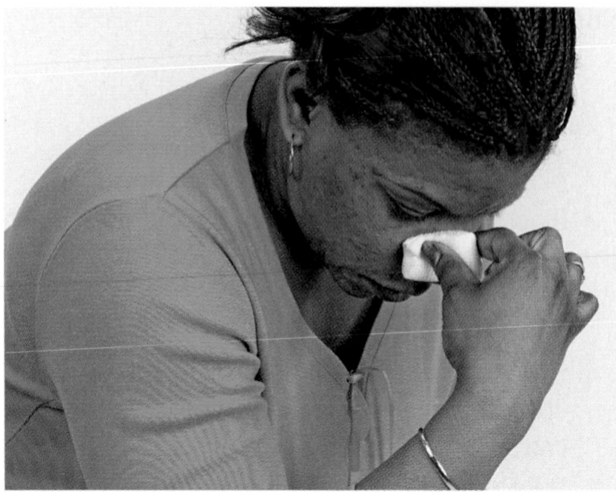

Figure 3-15 Pinch nostrils in soft area below the bridge of the nose.

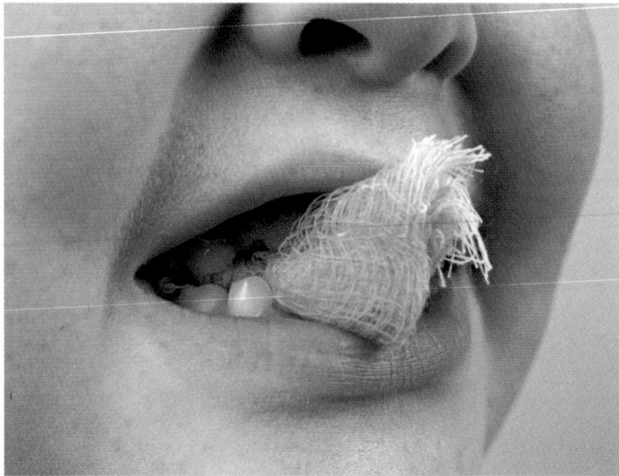

Figure 3-16 Stop bleeding with dressing over tooth socket.

Teeth and Mouth Injuries

For a tooth knocked out:

1. Have the victim sit with head tilted forward to let blood drain out.
2. To control bleeding, fold or roll gauze into a pad and place it over the tooth socket. Have victim bite down to put pressure on the area for 20 to 30 minutes (Figure 3-16).
3. Save the tooth, which may be reimplanted if the victim sees a dentist very soon. Touching only the tooth's crown, rinse it if dirty and replace it in its socket if possible; hold it in place with gauze pad. Otherwise, put it in a container of milk, the victim's saliva, or cool water.
4. Get the victim and the tooth to a dentist. (Most dentists have 24-hour emergency call numbers.)

For other bleeding in the mouth:

1. Have the victim sit with head tilted forward to let blood drain out.
2. **For a wound penetrating the lip:** Put a rolled dressing between the lip and the gum. Hold a second dressing against the outside lip.
3. For a bleeding tongue: Put a dressing on the wound and apply pressure.
4. Do not rinse the mouth (this may prevent clotting).
5. Do not let victim swallow blood, which may cause vomiting.
6. Tell the victim to not drink anything warm for several hours.
7. Seek medical attention if bleeding is severe or does not stop.

Bandages

Bandages are used for covering a dressing, keeping the dressing on a wound, and applying pressure to stop bleeding. Because only dressings touch the wound itself, bandages need to be clean but not necessarily sterile. As described in Chapter 7, bandages are also used to support or immobilize an injury to bones, joints, or muscles and to reduce swelling.

Types of Bandages

All the following are examples of bandages (Figure 3-17):

- Adhesive compresses or strips for small wounds that combine a dressing with an adhesive bandage
- Adhesive tape rolls (cloth, plastic, paper)
- Tubular bandages for finger or toe
- Elastic bandages
- Cloth roller bandages
- Triangular bandages (or folded square cloths)
- Any cloth or other material improvised to meet purposes of bandaging

Learning Checkpoint 3

1. Name one circumstance in which you might want to promote bleeding.

___

2. True or False: The first thing to do when you see an object impaled in a wound is to pull it out so that you can put direct pressure on the wound to stop the bleeding.
3. True or False: An amputated part should be kept cold but not put in direct contact with ice.
4. List two or three signs of a possible skull fracture. What is one thing you should not do to stop bleeding from the head if you suspect a skull fracture?

___

5. With an eye injury, why would you cover the uninjured eye too?

___

6. Describe three ways you can try to remove a small particle from the eye.

___

7. True or False: For bleeding from within the ear, roll a piece of gauze into a plug and try to seal the ear with it.
8. A nosebleed victim should first try to stop the bleeding by pinching the nostrils closed for ____ minutes. During this time, list two or three things the victim should not do.

___

9. True or False: A knocked-out tooth can be reimplanted if it is kept wet and the victim reaches a dentist soon.
10. True or False: Repeatedly rinsing the mouth with cool water is the best way to stop bleeding in the mouth.

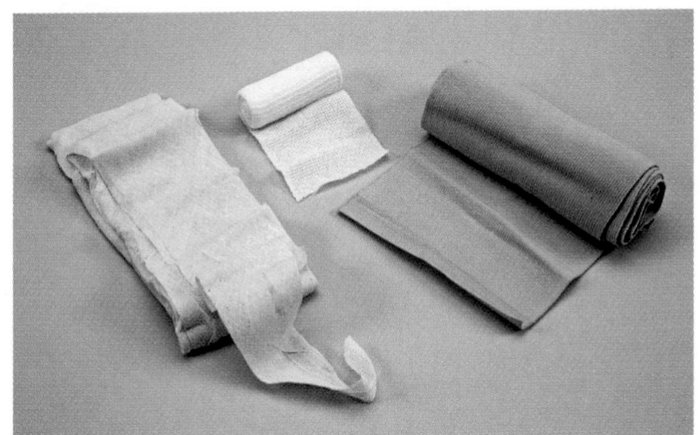

Figure 3-17 Types of bandages.

Follow these guidelines for bandaging:

1. To put pressure on a wound to stop bleeding or to prevent swelling of an injury, apply the bandage firmly—but not so tight that it cuts off circulation. With a bandage around a limb, check the fingers or toes for color, warmth, and sensation (normal touch, not tingling) to make sure circulation is not cut off. If there are signs of reduced circulation, unwrap the bandage and reapply it less tightly.
2. Since swelling continues after many injuries, keep checking the tightness of the bandage. Swelling may make a loose bandage tight enough to cut off circulation.
3. With a bandaged wound, be sure the bandage is secure enough that the dressing will not move and expose the wound to possible contamination.
4. With elastic and roller bandages, anchor the first end and tie, tape, or pin the ending section in place.

5. Use a nonelastic roller bandage to make a circular pressure bandage around a limb to control bleeding and protect the wound.
6. An elastic roller bandage is used to support a joint and prevent swelling. At the wrist or ankle a figure-eight wrap is used.

Internal Bleeding

Internal bleeding is any bleeding within the body in which the blood does not escape from an open wound. A closed wound may have minor local bleeding in the skin and other superficial tissue, causing a bruise. A more serious injury can cause deeper organs to bleed severely. This bleeding, although unseen, can be life threatening.

For simple closed wounds:

When You See

- Bruising
- Signs of pain

Do This First

1. Check for signs and symptoms of a fracture or sprain (see Chapter 7) and give appropriate first aid.
2. Put an ice or cold pack on the area to control bleeding, reduce swelling, and reduce pain.
3. With an arm or leg, wrap the area with an elastic bandage. Keep the part raised to help reduce swelling.

Additional Care

- Seek medical attention if you suspect a more serious injury such as a fracture or sprain

For internal bleeding:

When You See

- Abdomen is tender, swollen, bruised, or hard
- Blood vomited or coughed up, or present in urine
- Cool, clammy skin, may be pale or bluish
- Thirst
- Possible confusion, light-headedness

Do This First

1. Have the victim lie down on the back with feet raised about 12 inches.
2. Call 911.
3. Be alert for vomiting. Put a victim who vomits or becomes unresponsive in the recovery position.
4. Keep the victim from becoming chilled or overheated.

Additional Care

- Calm and reassure the victim
- If the victim becomes unresponsive, monitor the ABCs and give care as needed
- Treat for shock (see Chapter 4)

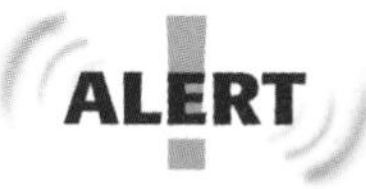

Internal Bleeding

Do not give the victims anything to drink even if they are very thirsty.

Learning Checkpoint 4

1. True or False: To control bleeding, make a pressure bandage as tight as you can get it.
2. You have put a roller bandage around a woman's arm to control bleeding from a laceration. A few minutes later she says her fingers are tingling. You feel her hand, and her fingers are cold. What should you do?

Perform the Skill

Applying a Circular Pressure Bandage

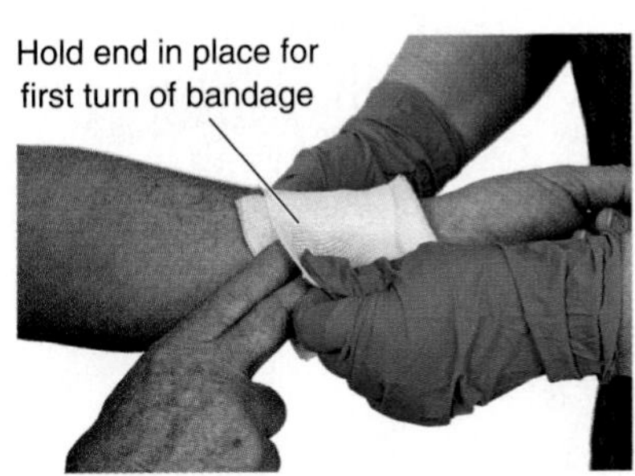

1 Anchor the starting end of the bandage below the wound dressing.

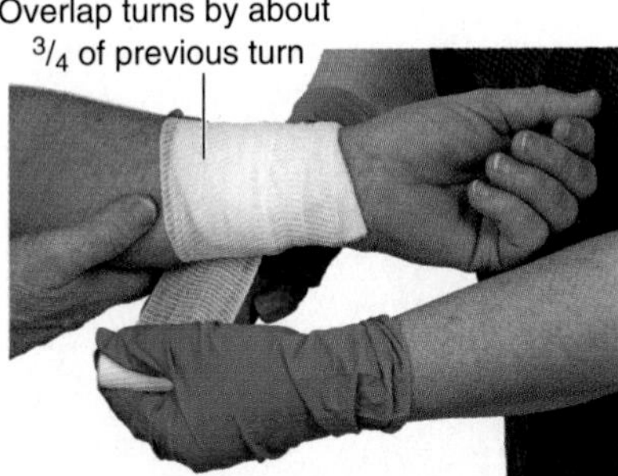

2 Make several circular turns, then overlap turns.

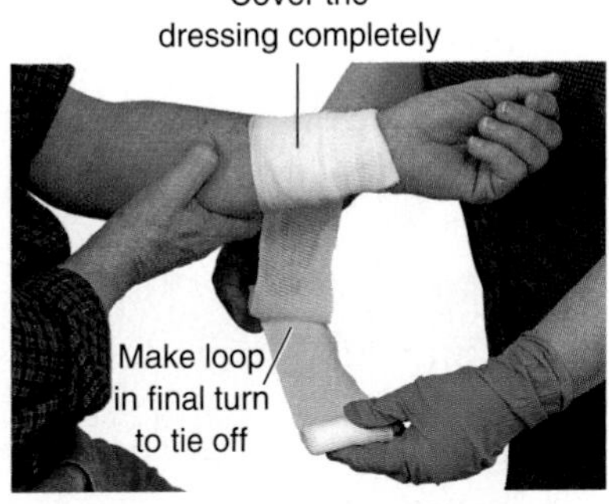

3 Work up the limb.

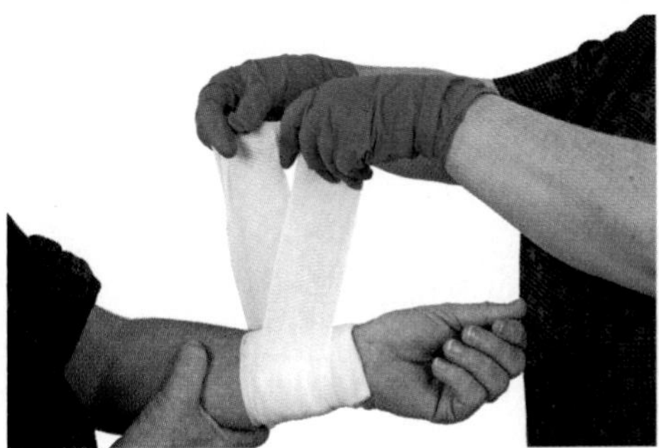

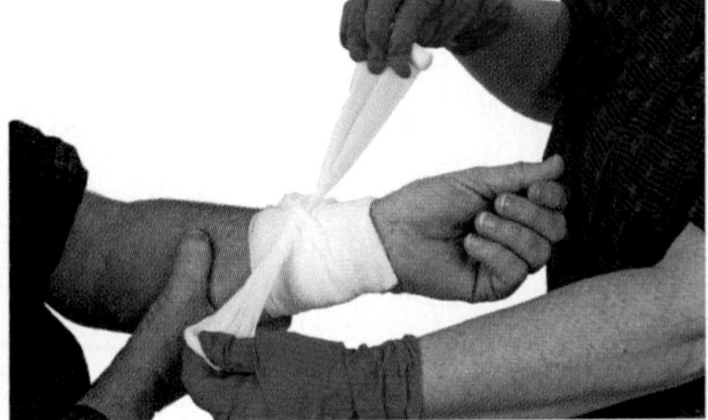

4 Tape or tie the end of the bandage in place.

3. When applying a bandage over a dressing, the bandage should:

_____ **a.** Hold down only the corners of the dressing so the wound can "breathe"

_____ **b.** Be soaked first in cold water

_____ **c.** Cover the entire dressing

_____ **d.** Be loose enough so it can be slid to one side to change the dressing

4. Name three ways you can secure the end of an elastic roller bandage.

____

Perform the Skill

Applying a Roller Bandage

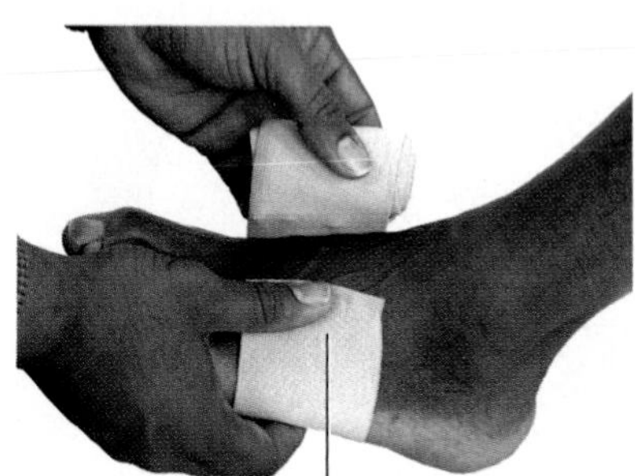

1 Anchor the starting end of the bandage.

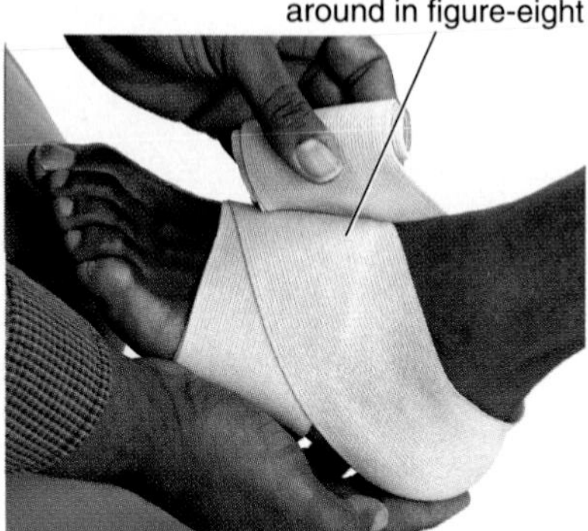

2 Turn bandage diagonally across top of foot and around ankle.

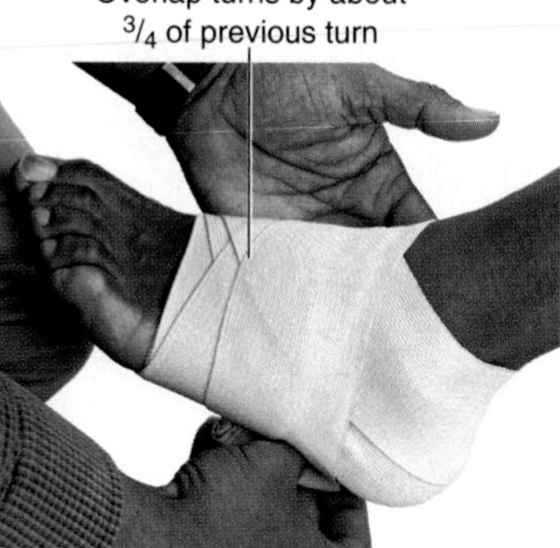

3 Continue with overlapping figure-eight turns.

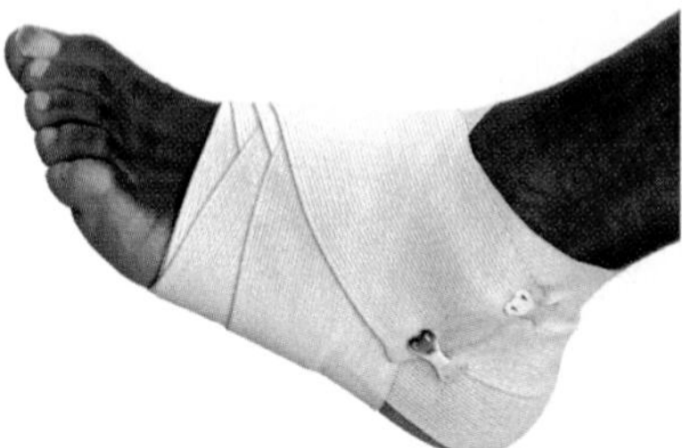

4 Fasten end of bandage with clips, tape, or safety pins.

Chapter

4 Shock

CHAPTER PREVIEW

Shock is a dangerous condition in which not enough oxygen-rich blood is reaching vital organs in the body. The brain, heart, and other organs need a continual supply of oxygen. Anything that happens to or in the body that significantly reduces blood flow can cause shock.

Shock is a life-threatening emergency. It may develop quickly or gradually. Always call 911 for a victim in shock.

CAUSES OF SHOCK

- *Severe bleeding* causes shock when there is not enough blood circulating in the body to bring required oxygen to vital organs. With internal injuries, it may not be obvious the victim is bleeding.
- *Heart problems*, like a heart attack or heart rhythm problem, cause shock when the heart cannot pump enough blood to meet the body's needs.
- *Nervous system injuries*, such as those caused by neck or spine injuries, can affect the heart or blood vessels in ways that prevent adequate blood from reaching vital organs.

Many other types of injuries can also cause some degree of shock. Some specific examples are as follows:

- Dehydration (such as may occur in heatstroke or with severe vomiting or diarrhea)
- Heart failure
- Serious infections
- Severe burns
- Allergic reactions (see later section on Anaphylaxis)

FIRST AID FOR SHOCK

Shock has various signs and symptoms depending on its cause and severity. A victim with any serious injury should be assumed to be at risk of shock, even if you do not see all these signs and symptoms (**Figure 4-1**).

When You See

- Anxiety, confusion, agitation, or restlessness
- Dizziness, light-headedness
- Cool, clammy or sweating, pale or bluish skin
- Rapid, shallow breathing
- Thirst
- Nausea, vomiting
- Changing levels of responsiveness

Do This First

1. Check the ABCs and care for life-threatening injuries.
2. Call 911.
3. Have the victim lie on his or her back and raise the legs about 8 to 12 inches (unless the victim may have a spine injury). Loosen any tight clothing (**Figure 4-2**).
4. Try to maintain the victim's normal body temperature. If lying on the ground, put a coat or blanket under the victim. If in doubt, keep the victim warm with a blanket or coat over the victim (**Figure 4-3**).

Additional Care

- Stay with the victim and offer reassurance and comfort

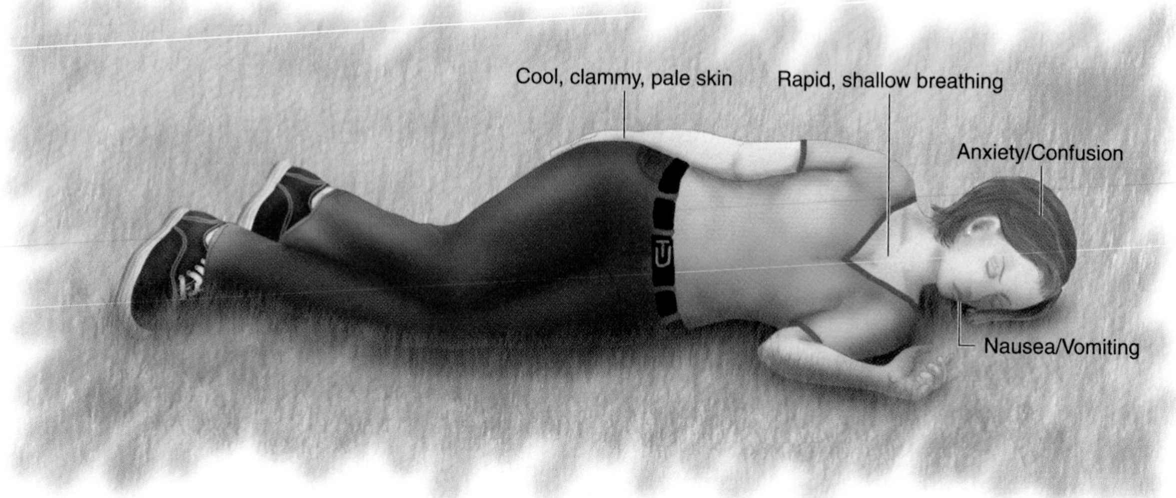

Figure 4-1 The signs and symptoms of shock.

- Put an unresponsive victim (if no suspected spinal injury) in the recovery position
- Keep bystanders from crowding around the victim

Anaphylaxis

Anaphylaxis is a severe allergic reaction, also called anaphylactic shock. It is a life-threatening emergency because the victim's airway may swell, making breathing difficult or impossible. Always call 911 for an anaphylaxis emergency.

Common causes of anaphylaxis include:

- Certain drugs (such as penicillins, sulfa)
- Certain foods (such as peanuts, shellfish, eggs)
- Insect stings and bites (such as bees or wasps)

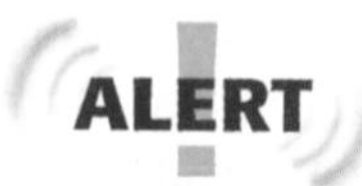

Shock

Do not let a shock victim eat, drink, or smoke. Note that sweating in a shock victim is not necessarily a sign of being too warm. If in doubt, it is better to ensure a shock victim's body temperature by keeping the victim warm.

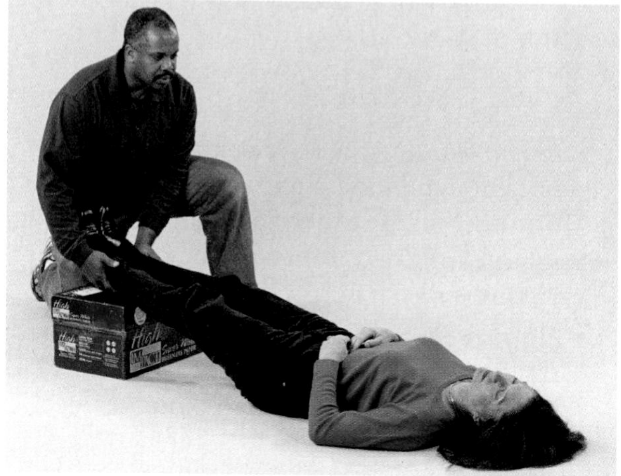

Figure 4-2 Raise the legs of a shock victim.

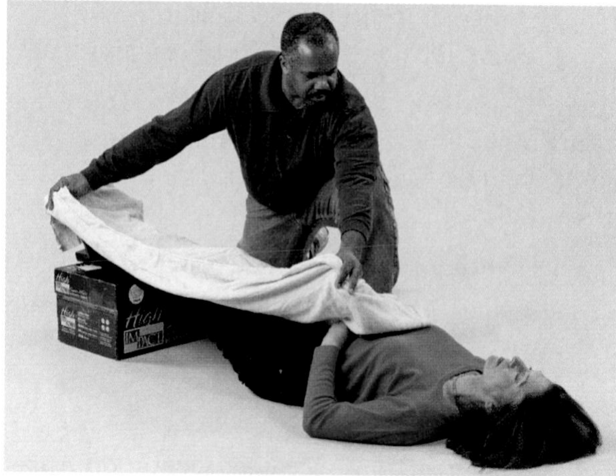

Figure 4-3 Help maintain the victim's normal body temperature.

Learning Checkpoint 1

1. True or False: Because a shock victim is thirsty and may be dehydrated, offer clear fluids to drink.

2. True or False: A spinal injury can cause shock.

3. Which of these actions should you take *first* for a victim in shock because of external bleeding?

a. Stop the bleeding

b. Raise the legs

c. Loosen constricting clothing

d. Cover the victim with a blanket

4. A shock victim is likely to have which signs and symptoms?

a. Vomiting, diarrhea, red blotchy face

b. Nausea, thirst, clammy skin

c. Incontinence, hives, swollen legs

d. Headache, painful abdomen, coughing

5. What is the most important action to take for *all shock victims?*

____

Some people who know they have a severe allergy may carry an emergency epinephrine kit such as an EpiPen®. This medication can stop the anaphylactic reaction. Ask a victim about this and help him or her open and use the kit as needed. (The EpiPen® is removed from its case and the cap removed. The tip is then jabbed into the muscle of the outer part of the thigh and held there 5–10 seconds [**Figure 4-4**]. The injection site is then massaged for a few seconds). The effects of the emergency epinephrine will last 15–20 minutes.

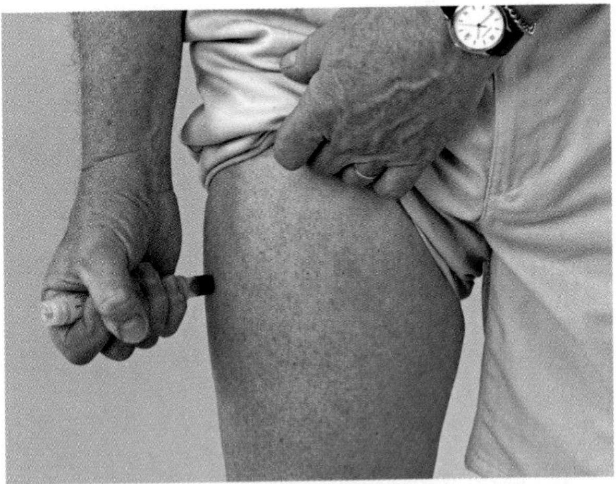

Figure 4-4 Position the EpiPen® firmly against the thigh to inject.

When You See

- Difficulty breathing, wheezing
- Complaints of tightness in throat or chest
- Swelling of the face and neck, puffy eyes
- Anxiety, agitation
- Nausea, vomiting
- Changing responsiveness

Do This First

1. Call 911.
2. Check the ABCs and give care as needed.
3. Help victim use his or her epinephrine kit.
4. Help victim sit up in position of easiest breathing (Figure 4-5).

Additional Care

- Stay with the victim and offer reassurance and comfort
- Put an unresponsive victim (if no suspected spinal injury) in the recovery position

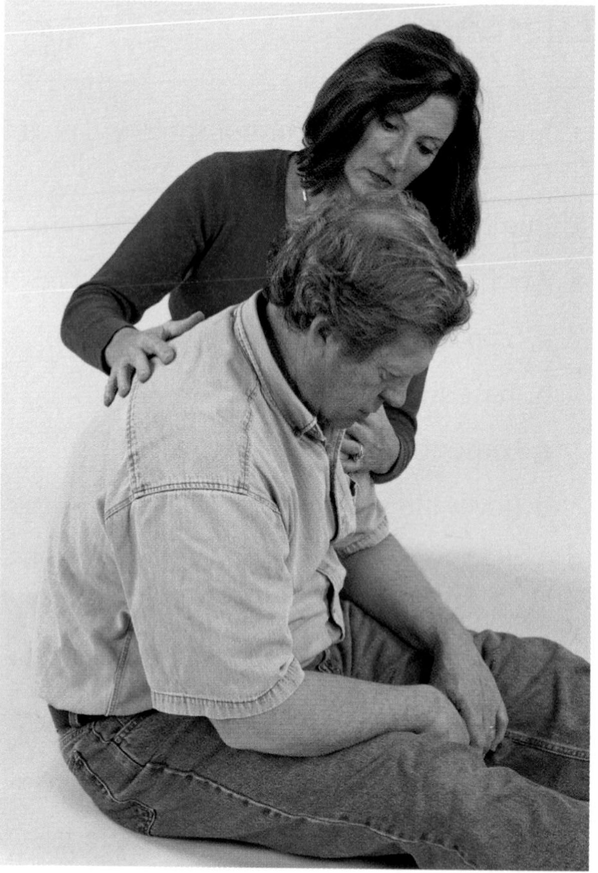

Figure 4-5 Assist an anaphylaxis victim to the position of easiest breathing.

Learning Checkpoint 2

1. True or False: Ask a victim having an anaphylactic reaction about any allergies.
2. True or False: A bee sting can cause a severe allergic reaction.
3. The major risk for a victim in anaphylaxis is:
   - **a.** Swelling around the eyes
   - **b.** Heart attack
   - **c.** Internal bleeding
   - **d.** Breathing problems
4. How should a victim in anaphylaxis be positioned if having trouble breathing?

____

Chapter

5 Burns

CHAPTER PREVIEW

- Heat Burns
- How Bad Is the Burn?
- Smoke Inhalation
- Chemical Burns
- Electrical Burns and Shocks

Burns of the skin or deeper tissues may be caused by heat, chemicals, or electricity. Mild heat burns and sunburn may need only simple first aid, but severe burns can be a medical emergency.

HEAT BURNS

Heat burns may be caused by flames or contact with steam or any hot object. The severity of a burn depends on the amount of damage to the skin and other tissues under the skin.

Put Out the Fire!

If the victim's clothing is on fire, have the victim **stop, drop, and roll.** Use water to put out any flames. Even when the fire is out, the skin will keep burning if it is still hot, so cool the burn area with water immediately, except with very severe burns. Also remove the victim's clothing and jewelry, if possible without further injuring the victim, because they may still be hot and continue to burn the victim.

How Bad Is the Burn?

- **First-degree burns** (also called superficial burns) damage only the skin's outer layer, like a typical sunburn. These are minor burns and usually heal by themselves.
- **Second-degree burns** (also called partial-thickness burns) damage the skin's deeper layers. When small they may not be too serious, but larger second-degree burns require medical attention.
- **Third-degree burns** (also called full-thickness burns) damage the skin all the way through and may burn the muscle or other tissues. These are medical emergencies (Figure 5-1).

Also important is the location of the burn on the body. Burns on the face, genitals, or hands or feet are more serious and require medical care.

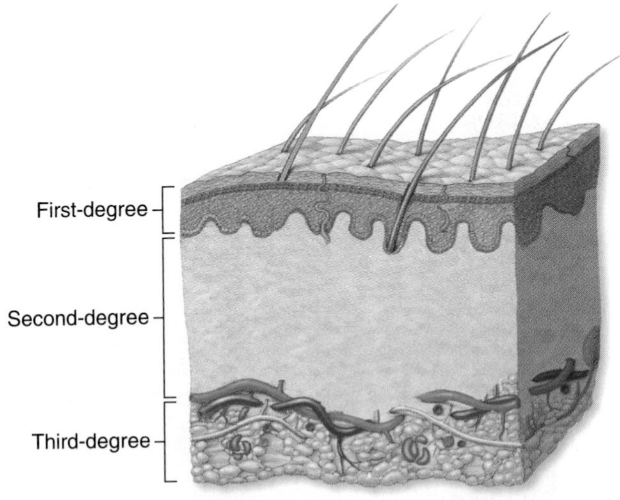

Figure 5-1 Burn depth.

First-Degree Burns

When You See

- Skin is red, dry, and painful (Figure 5-2)
- May be some swelling
- Skin not broken

Do This First

1. Stop the burning by removing the heat source.
2. Cool the burned area with room temperature water. Immerse a small area in a sink or bucket, or cover a larger area with wet cloth for at least 10 minutes–but not most of the body.
3. Remove clothing and jewelry or any other constricting item before the area swells.
4. Protect the burn from friction or pressure.

Additional Care

- Aloe vera gel can be used on the skin for comfort

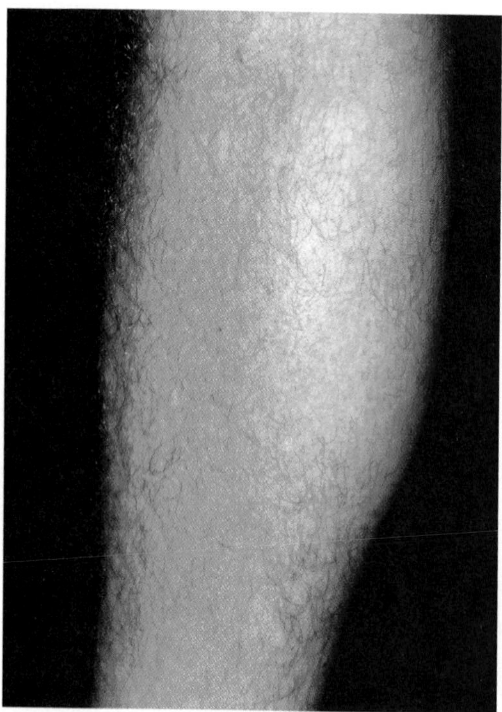

Figure 5-2 First-degree burn.

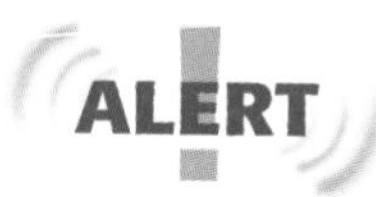

Burn

Do not put butter on a burn.
Do not use icy or cold water on a burn because even though it may relieve pain, the cold can actually cause additional damage to the skin.

PREVENTING SUNBURN

Skin cancer, now the most common cancer in the U.S., is usually caused by exposure to the sun. People who work outside are especially vulnerable to skin cancer. Each year 40,000 cases of melanoma, the deadliest skin cancer, occur in the U.S. Preventing frequent sunburn helps prevent this cancer:

- Avoid exposure to the midday sun
- Wear a wide-brimmed hat and protective clothing
- Use SPF 35 sunscreen or sunblock applied 20 minutes before sun exposure and at least every 2 hours

Second-Degree Burns

When You See

- Skin is swollen and red, may be blotchy or streaked (Figure 5-3)
- Blisters that may be weeping clear fluid
- Signs of significant pain

Do This First

1. Stop the burning by removing the heat source.
2. Cool the burned area with room temperature water. Immerse a small area in a sink or bucket, or cover a larger area (but not most of the body) with wet cloth for at least 10 minutes or until the area is free of pain even after removal from the water (Figure 5-4).
3. Remove clothing and jewelry from the area before the area swells.

4. Put a dressing over the burn to protect the area, but keep it loose and do not tape it to the skin (Figure 5-5).

Additional Care

- For large burns or burns on the face, genitals, hands or feet, seek medical attention

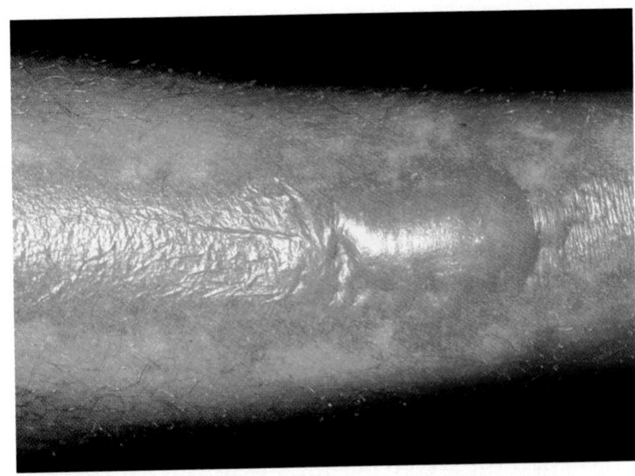

Figure 5-3 Second-degree burn.

Burn

Do not break skin blisters! This could cause an infection. Be gentle when covering the area.

Third-Degree Burns

When You See

- Skin damage, charred skin, or white leathery skin (Figure 5-6)
- May have signs and symptoms of shock (pale, clammy skin; nausea and vomiting; fast breathing)

Do This First

1. Stop the burning by removing the heat source.
2. Cool surrounding first- and second-degree burns only.
3. Remove clothing and jewelry before the area swells.
4. Call 911.
5. Prevent shock: have the victim lie down, elevate the legs, and maintain normal body temperature.
6. Carefully cover the burn with a dressing. Do not apply a cream or ointment.

Additional Care

- Monitor the victim's ABCs and give care as needed

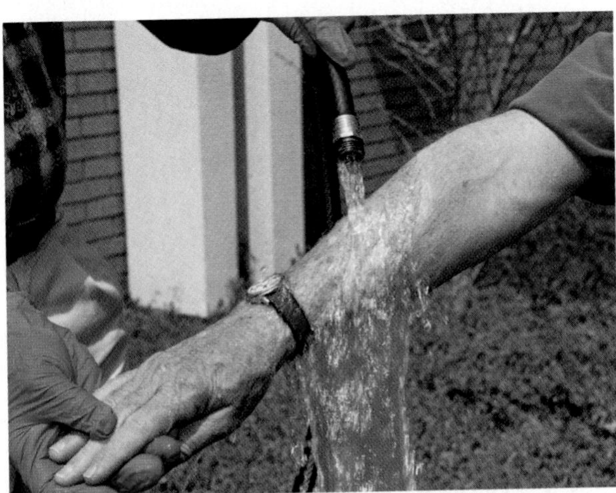

Figure 5-4 Cool a small burned area with water.

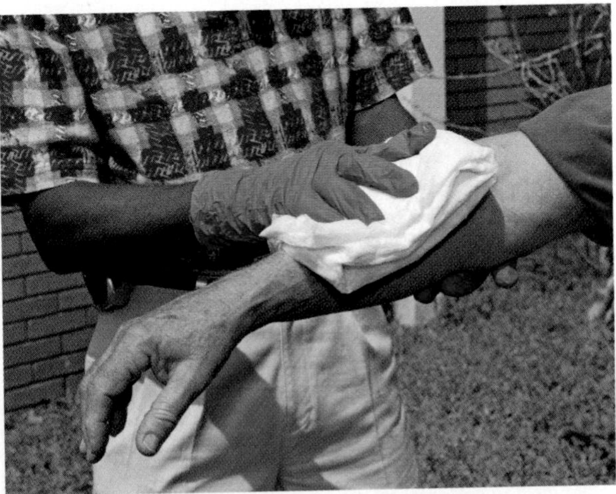

Figure 5-5 Cover the burn with a dressing.

Learning Checkpoint 1

1. True or False: With a victim with a second-degree burn, you should break skin blisters before covering the area with a burn treatment ointment to help it work faster.
2. With a victim with a third-degree burn, you should cool only a ________ area with water because of the risk of shock or hypothermia.
3. As you are leaving work, you see a man working on his car in the parking lot. He suddenly screams and backs away, his clothing on fire. What do you do? List in correct order the first four actions you should take.

____

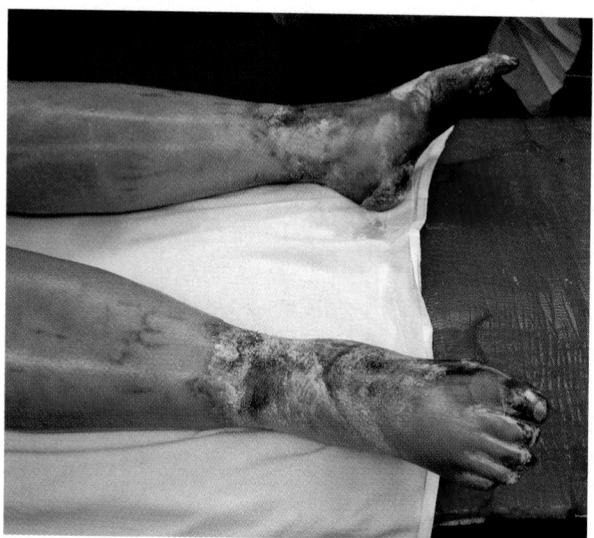

Figure 5-6 Third-degree burn.

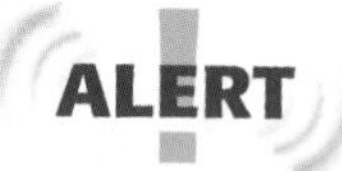

Third-Degree Burn

With third-degree burns do not cool more than 20% of the body with water (10% for a child) because of the risk of hypothermia and shock. Do not touch the burn or put anything on it. Do not give the victim anything to drink.

Smoke Inhalation

Inhaling very hot air or smoke can burn the airway from the mouth to the lungs. This can be a medical emergency. It is important to note that symptoms from smoke inhalation may not become obvious for up to 48 hours after exposure.

When You See

- Smoke visible in area
- Coughing, wheezing, hoarse voice
- Possible burned area on face or chest
- Difficulty breathing

Do This First

1. Get the victim to fresh air, or fresh air to the victim.
2. Call 911.
3. Help the victim into a position for easy breathing.

Additional Care

- Put an unresponsive victim in the recovery position
- Monitor the victim's ABCs and give care as needed

Chemical Burns

Many strong chemicals found in workplaces and the home can "burn" the skin on contact (**Figure 5-7**). Sometimes the burn develops slowly and in some cases the victim may not be aware of the burn for up to 24 hours. Both acids and alkalis, and liquids and solids can cause serious burns. Since the chemical reaction can continue as long as the substance is on the skin, you must flush it off with water as soon as possible.

When You See

- A chemical on the victim's skin or clothing
- Complaints of pain or a burning sensation
- A spilled substance on or around an unresponsive victim
- A smell of fumes in the air

Do This First

1. With a dry chemical, first brush it off the victim's skin (Figure 5-8). (Wear medical exam gloves to avoid contact with the substance yourself.)
2. With a spilled liquid giving off fumes, move the victim or ventilate the area.
3. Wash off the area as quickly as possible with running water for 20 to 30 minutes. Use a sink, hose, or even a shower to flush the whole area of contact (Figure 5-9).
4. Remove clothing and jewelry from the burn area (Figure 5-10).
5. Call 911 for any chemical burn.

Additional Care

- If chemicals were spilled in a confined area, leave the area with the victim because of the risk of fumes
- Put a dry dressing over the burn (Figure 5-11)
- Seek medical attention for any chemical burn

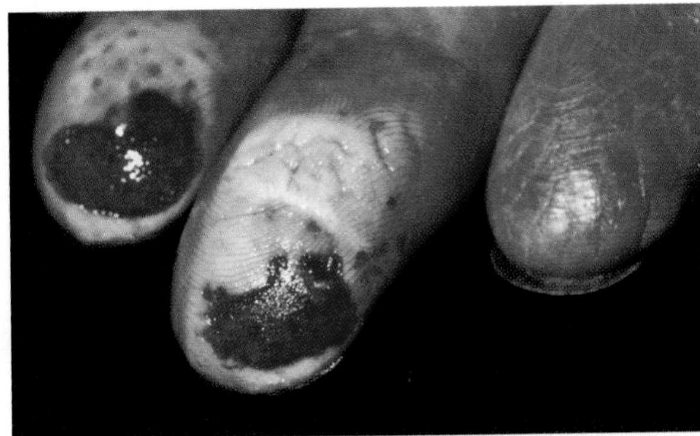

Figure 5-7 A chemical burn.

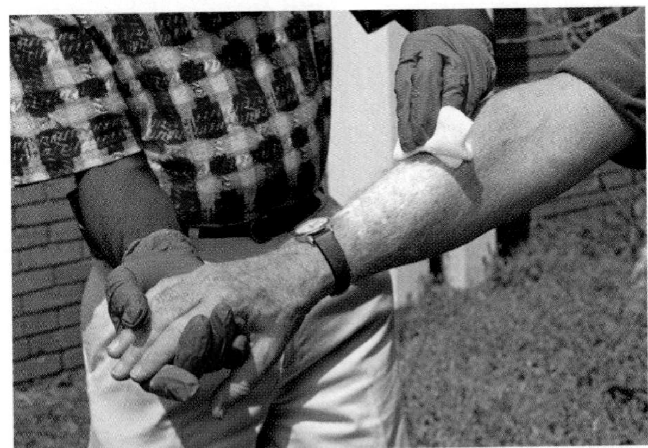

Figure 5-8 Brush a dry chemical from the skin.

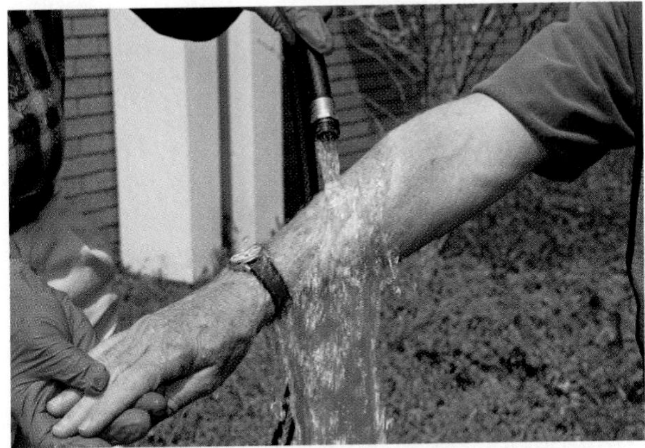

Figure 5-9 Flush the burned area with water.

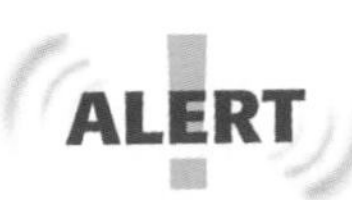

Chemical in the Eyes

With a chemical splashed in the eye, flush immediately with running water and continue for 20 minutes. Have the victim remove contact lenses. Tilt the victim's head so that the water runs away from the face and not into the other eye. After flushing, have the victim hold a dressing over the eye until a healthcare provider is seen.

Learning Checkpoint 2

1. A coworker has splashed an unknown liquid in her eye and is holding her hand over the eye. What should you do first?
   - a. Have her keep holding the eye closed so that her tears will wash out the chemical
   - b. Call 911 and wait for healthcare personnel to take care of her eye
   - c. Immediately flush the eye with running water
   - d. Mix baking soda with water and pour it into her eye
2. Describe the first action to take if a victim has a dry chemical on the skin.

   ____

3. You enter a storage room and find an unresponsive man lying on the floor. Beside him is an open jug and a puddle of a dark liquid. There's a strong smell in the air. What do you do?

   ____

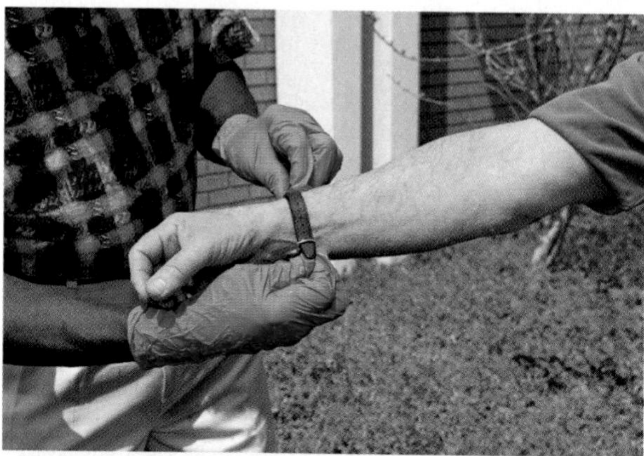

Figure 5-10 Remove clothing and jewelry.

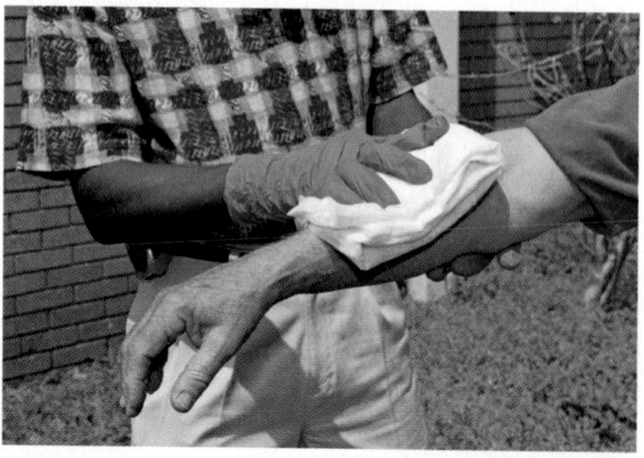

Figure 5-11 Put a dry dressing over the burn.

Electrical Burns and Shocks

Electrical burns may include:

- External burns caused by the heat of electricity
- Electrical injuries caused by electricity flowing through the body

External burns resulting from heat or flames caused by electricity are cared for the same as heat burns. Electrical injuries may cause only minor external burns where the electricity both entered and left the body (called entrance and exit wounds) (**Figure 5-12**). But electricity flowing through the body can stop the victim's heart and cause other serious injuries.

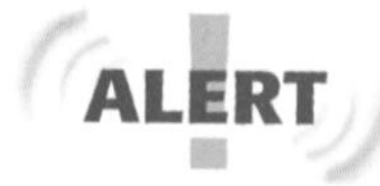

Electrical Shock

Do not touch a victim you think has had an electrical shock! First make sure the power is turned off or the person is well away from the power source. Turn off the circuit breaker and call 911.

Note that electrical burns can cause massive internal injuries even when the external burn may look minor.

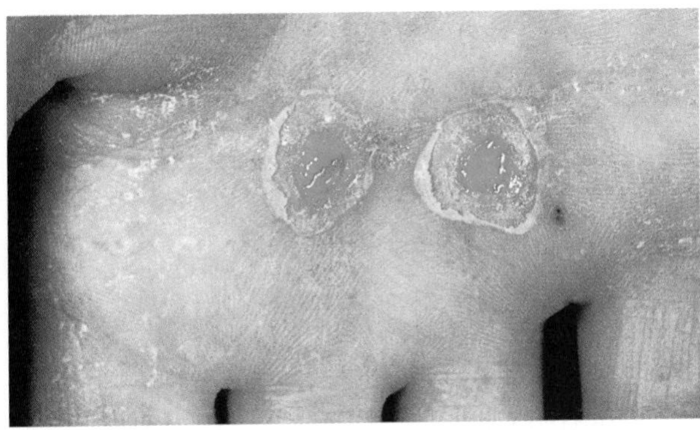

Figure 5-12 An electrical burn.

When You See

- A source of electricity near the victim: bare wires, power cords, an electrical device
- Burned area of skin, possibly both entrance and exit wounds
- Changing levels of responsiveness

Do This First

1. Do not touch the victim until you know the area is safe. Unplug or turn off the power.
2. With an unresponsive victim, check the victim's ABCs and give care as needed.
3. Call 911.
4. Care for the burn (stop the burning, cool the area, remove clothing and jewelry, cover the burn).
5. Prevent shock by having the victim lie down, elevating the legs, and maintaining normal body temperature.

Additional Care

- Keep an unresponsive victim in the recovery position and monitor the ABCs until help arrives

HIGH POWER LINES

If a power line is down, do not approach a victim in contact with the line. Call 911 immediately. Do not try to move the wire away using any object. Wait for emergency workers to arrive, and keep others away from the scene.

LIGHTNING STRIKES

Lightning strikes often cause serious injury. In addition to burns, the electrical shock may affect the heart and brain and cause temporary blindness or deafness, unresponsiveness or seizures, bleeding, bone fractures, and cardiac arrest. Call 911 immediately and give basic life support care, treating the most serious injuries first.

Learning Checkpoint 3

1. True or False: The first thing to do for an unresponsive victim in contact with an electrical wire is pour water over the area of contact.
2. What is the safest way to stop the electricity when someone is shocked by an electrical appliance? How should you not try to stop it?

____

3. Driving home from work, you are stopped behind a car that has struck a telephone pole. You get out to help the driver and see a power line dangling from the pole in contact with the roof of the car. Your first action should be to:
   - a. Use your cell phone to call 911
   - b. Look for a stick or piece of wood to push the wire away from the car
   - c. Try to pull the victim out the car window
   - d. Give any needed first aid by leaning in the car window

Chapter

6 Serious Injuries

CHAPTER PREVIEW

- Head and Spinal Injuries
- Chest Injuries
- Abdominal Injuries
- Pelvic Injuries

Many factors affect how serious an injury is. As you have learned, injuries that threaten the victim's airway, breathing, or circulation are life threatening. Severe bleeding is also very serious. This chapter describes some additional injuries in specific areas of the body that can be very serious and may become life threatening.

HEAD AND SPINAL INJURIES

Any injury to the head may also injure the spine. Whenever you find a serious head injury, suspect a neck or back injury also.

Skull Fractures

A skull fracture is life threatening. Call 911 immediately. Chapter 3, Bleeding and Wound Care, describes the signs and symptoms of a skull fracture and the first aid to give while waiting for help.

Brain Injuries

Brain injuries include bleeding, swelling, and concussion. A **concussion** is a temporary impairment of brain function and usually does not involve permanent damage. However, it is generally difficult to determine whether a victim's injury is moderately or very serious, and the victim may have a variety of signs and symptoms. Do not worry about trying to figure out what specifically is wrong—just call 911 and give supportive care while waiting for help.

When You See

- Head wound suggesting there was a blow to the head
- Changing levels of responsiveness, drowsiness
- Confusion, disorientation, memory loss about the injury
- Headache
- Dizziness
- Nausea, vomiting
- Unequal pupils

Do This First

For a responsive victim:

1. Have the victim lie down.
2. Keep the victim still and protect from becoming chilled or overheated.
3. Call 911 and monitor the victim's condition until help arrives.

For an unresponsive victim:

1. Check the victim's ABCs without moving the victim unless necessary. Assume there may be a spinal injury.
2. Control serious bleeding and cover any wounds with a dressing.
3. Call 911.
4. If the victim vomits, move him or her into the recovery position. If you suspect a spinal injury, support the head and neck at all times (Figure 6-1).

Additional Care

- Support the neck, even in a responsive victim, if you suspect a spinal injury

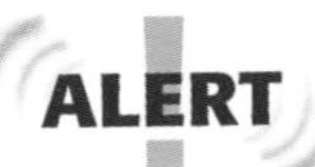

Brain Injury

Do not let the victim eat or drink anything. In some cases after a blow to the head the victim does not have the signs and symptoms listed earlier and does not seek medical care. Signs and symptoms appearing within 48 hours may indicate a more serious injury, however, including nausea and vomiting, severe or persistent headache, changing levels of responsiveness, problems with vision or speech, or seizures. Seek medical attention immediately if any of these occur following a head injury.

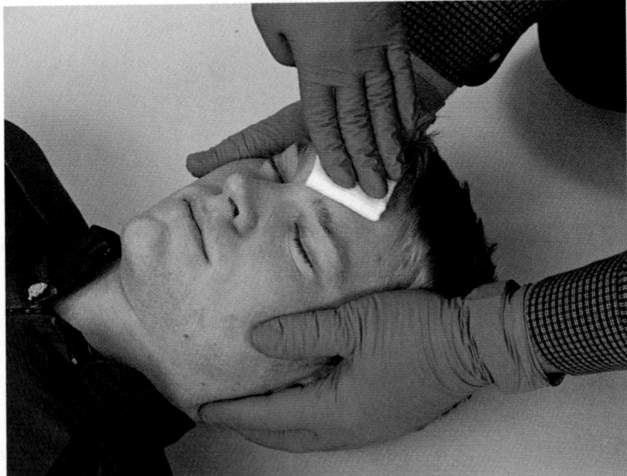

Figure 6-1 Support head in line with body for suspected spinal injury.

Spinal Injuries

A fracture of the neck or back is a spinal injury. This injury may be life threatening and can cause permanent paralysis. It is very important not to move the victim any more than necessary and to support the head and neck to prevent worsening the injury.

Suspect a spinal injury in these situations:

- A fall from a height (even a short height)
- A motor vehicle crash
- A blow to the head or back
- A crushing injury of the head, neck, or back
- A diving injury

When You See

For a responsive victim:

- Inability to move any body part
- Lack of sensation or tingling in hands or feet
- Deformed neck or back
- Breathing problems
- Headache

For an unresponsive victim:

- Deformed neck or back
- Signs of blow to head or back
- Nature of the emergency suggests possible spinal injury

Perform the Skill

Inline Stabilization

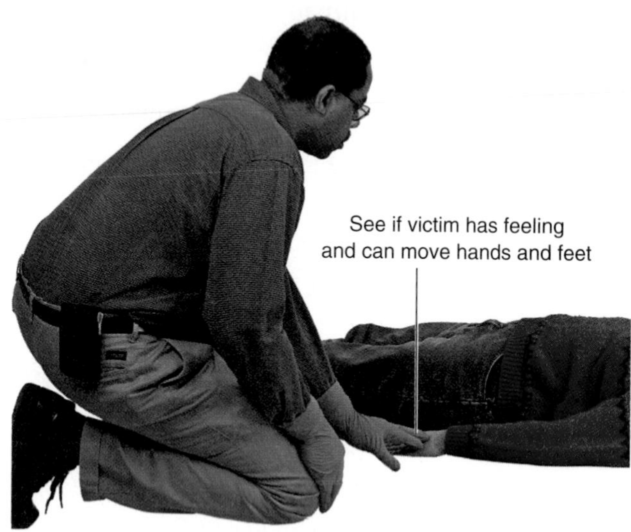
See if victim has feeling
and can move hands and feet

1 Assess a responsive victim for spinal injury.

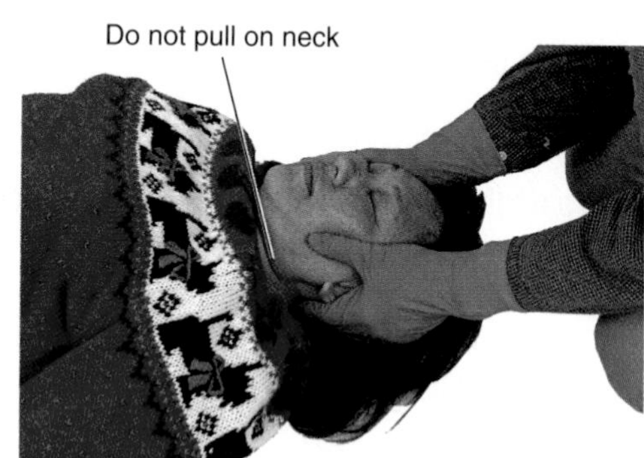
Do not pull on neck

2 Hold the victim's head with both hands to prevent movement of neck or spine.

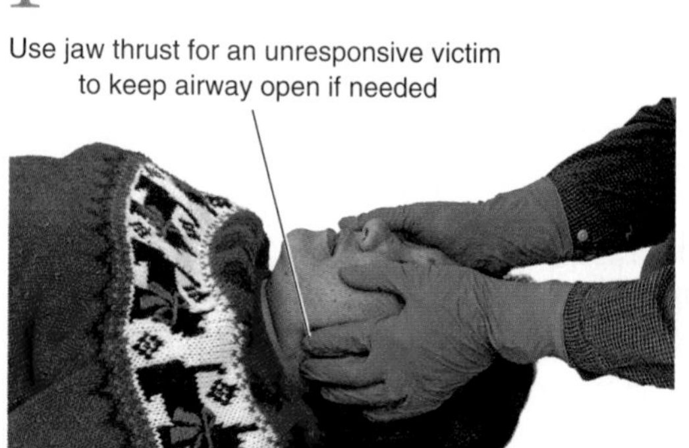
Use jaw thrust for an unresponsive victim
to keep airway open if needed

3 Monitor the ABCs.

4 Have someone call 911.

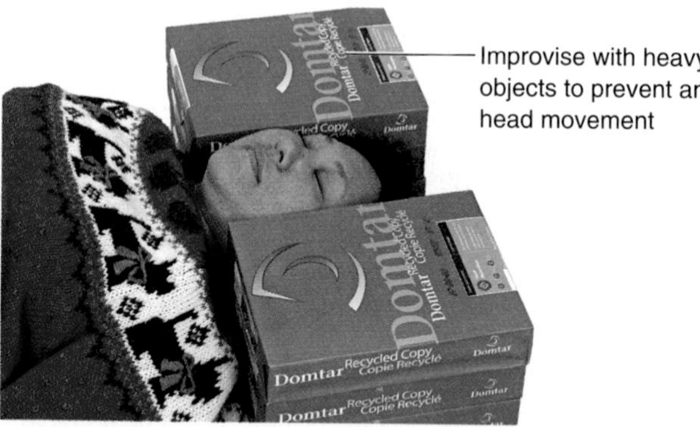
Improvise with heavy
objects to prevent any
head movement
Domtar
Domtar Recycled Copy Copie Recyclé

5 Use objects to maintain head support.

Perform the Skill

Rolling a Victim with Spinal Injury (Log Roll)

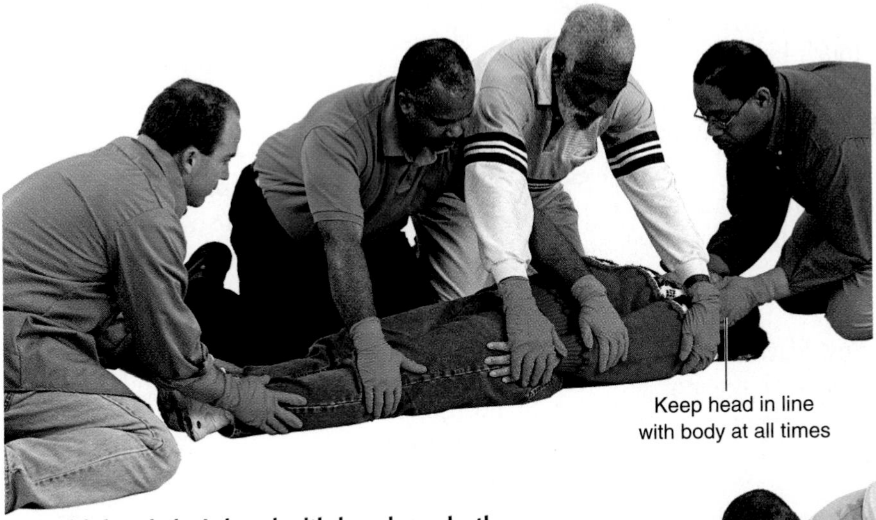

Keep head in line with body at all times

1 Hold the victim's head with hands on both sides over ears.

2 The first aider at the victim's head directs others to roll body as a unit.

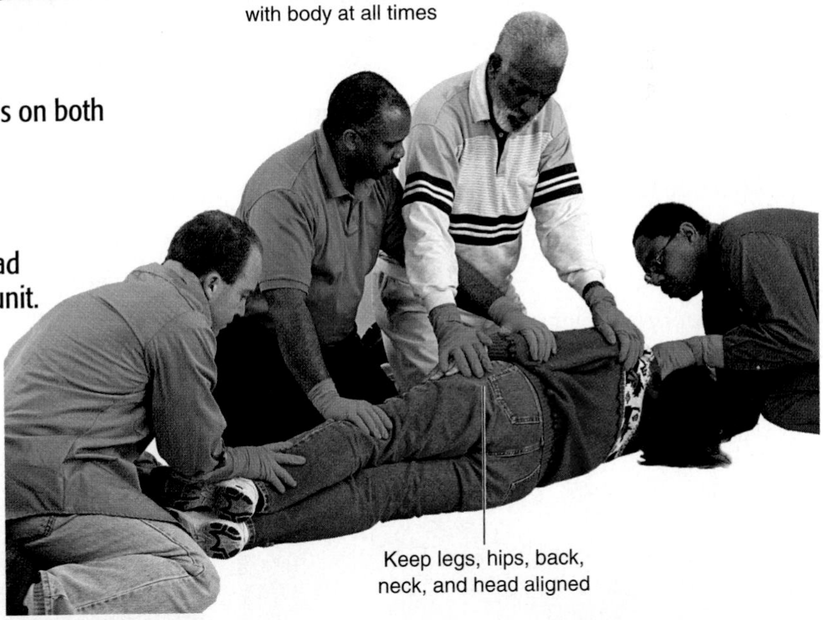

Keep legs, hips, back, neck, and head aligned

3 Continue to support head in new position on side.

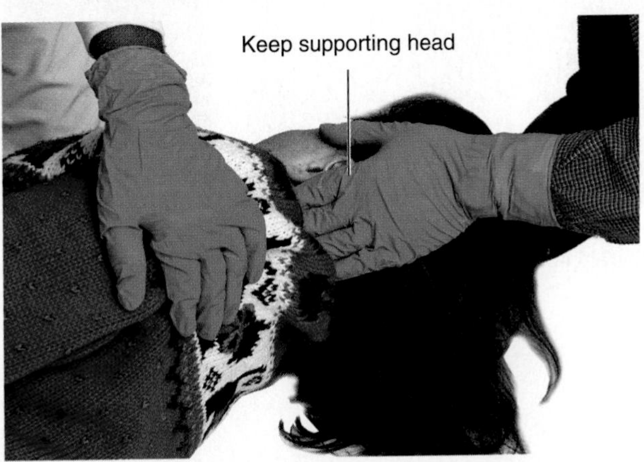

Do This First

1. Assess a responsive victim:
   - Can the victim move his or her fingers and toes?
   - Can the victim feel you touch his or her hands and feet?
2. Stabilize the victim's head and neck in the position found (Figure 6-2).
3. Monitor the ABCs. Use the jaw thrust to keep airway open if necessary in an unresponsive victim.
4. Send someone to call 911.
5. For a long wait, or if you must leave the victim to call 911, use padding or heavy objects on both sides of head to prevent movement.

Additional Care

- Reassure a responsive victim and tell him or her not to move
- Continue to monitor the ABCs until help arrives

Always support the victim's head and neck in the position found. Move the victim only if absolutely necessary, such as if a victim lying on his or her back vomits. If this occurs you must roll the victim on his or her side to let the mouth drain and allow breathing. The help of two or three others is necessary to keep the back and neck aligned during the move.

Chest Injuries

Serious chest injuries include broken ribs, objects impaled in the chest, and sucking chest wounds in which air passes in and out of the chest cavity. These wounds can be life threatening if breathing is affected. Chest injuries may result from such things as:

- Striking the steering wheel in a motor vehicle crash
- A blow to the chest
- A fall from a height

The general signs and symptoms of a chest injury include:

- Breathing problems
- Severe pain
- Deformity of the chest
- Possibly coughing blood

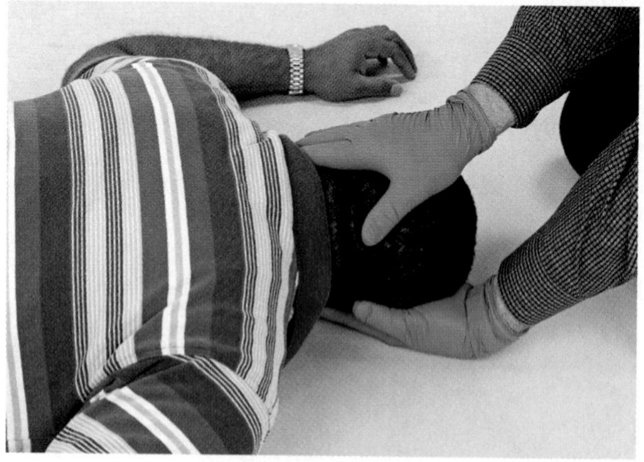

Figure 6-2 Support the head in the position you find the victim.

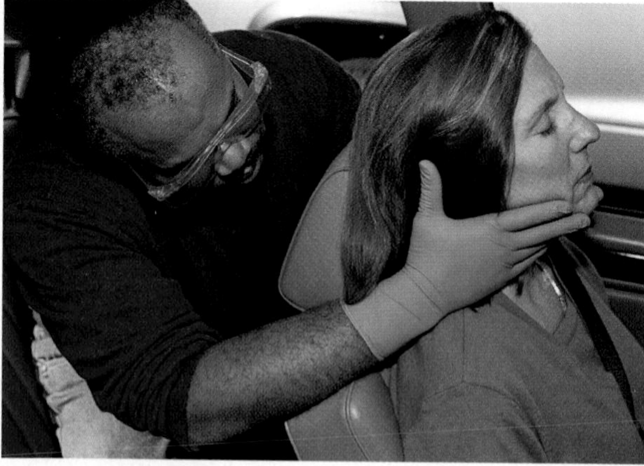

Learning Checkpoint 1

1. True or False: Suspect a spinal injury in any victim with a serious head injury.

2. True or False: You can easily tell a mild concussion from a serious brain injury by the signs and symptoms.

3. Check off the possible signs and symptoms of a brain injury:

_____ Headache

_____ Rapid blinking

_____ Memory loss

_____ Fingernail beds look blue

_____ Dizziness or confusion

_____ Nausea and vomiting

4. For an unresponsive victim you suspect may have a spinal injury:

a. First place victim on his or her back

b. Check the ABCs in the position in which you found the victim

c. Turn the head to one side in case the victim vomits

d. Move all body parts to see if anything feels broken

5. A spinal injury is likely in which of these situations? (Check all that apply.)

_____ The victim fell from a roof 20 feet high

_____ A victim with diabetes passes out at lunch

_____ The victim was in a car that hit a telephone pole

_____ A piece of heavy equipment fell from a shelf on the victim's head

_____ You find a victim slumped over in a desk chair

6. Which of these are signs and symptoms of a spinal injury? (Check all that apply.)

_____ Victim cannot stop coughing

_____ Victim's hands are tingling

_____ Victim has breathing problem

_____ Victim's face is bright red

_____ Unresponsive victim has nosebleed

_____ Victim's neck seems oddly turned

7. When do you call 911 for a victim with a potential spinal injury?

a. Call for all victims with potential spinal injury

b. Call only if the victim is unresponsive

c. Call for a responsive victim only if feeling is lost on one side of the victim

d. Call after waiting 10 minutes to see if an unresponsive victim awakes

8. In what position do you stabilize the head of a victim with a suspected spinal injury?

____

9. Roll a victim with a spinal injury onto his or her side only if the victim ______________.

10. In the company parking lot you see a car skid on an icy patch and smash into another car. The driver is still behind the wheel and looks dazed. Her forehead is bleeding. You ask her how she feels and she does not answer but just stares ahead. What should you do?

____

Broken Ribs

When You See

- Signs of pain with deep breathing or movement
- Victim holding ribs
- Shallow breathing

Do This First

1. Have person sit in position of easiest breathing.
2. Support the ribs with a pillow or soft padding loosely bandaged over the area and under the arm (Figure 6-3).
3. Call 911.

Additional Care

- Monitor the victim's breathing while waiting for help
- If needed, immobilize the arm with a sling and binder (see Chapter 7) to prevent movement and ease pain

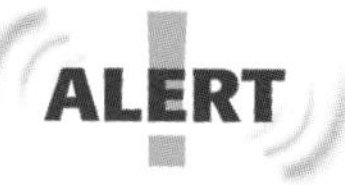

Chest Injury

Do not give the victim anything to eat or drink.

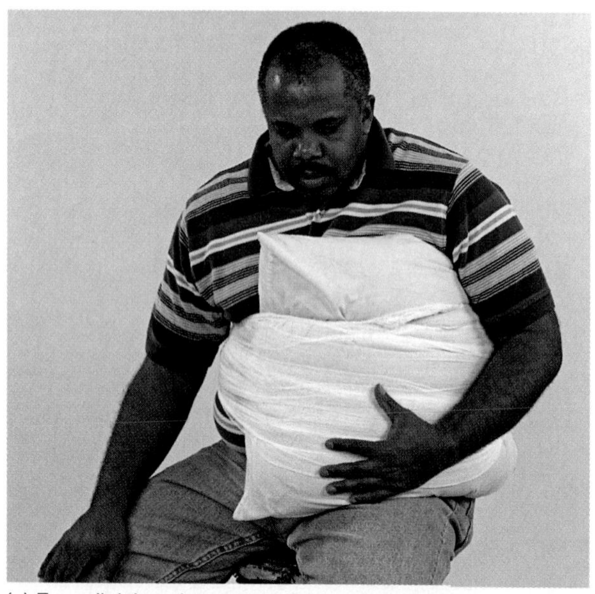

(a) For a rib injury do not wrap the bandage tightly.

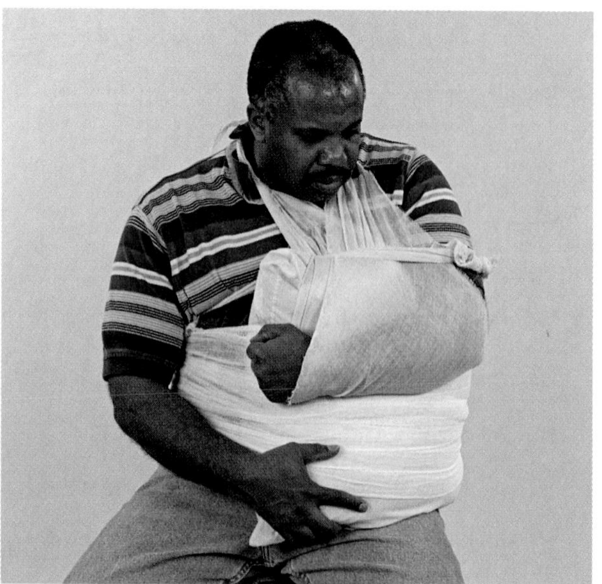

(b) Immobilizing the arm prevents movement of rib area.

Figure 6-3 Immobilize a rib injury.

Impaled Object

Removing an impaled object from the chest could cause additional bleeding and breathing problems. If a victim has an impaled object, it is important to leave it in place and seek medical attention.

When You See

- An object impaled in a chest wound

Do This First

1. Keep victim still. Victim may be seated or lying down.
2. Use bulky dressings or cloth to stabilize the object.
3. Bandage the area around the object (Figure 6-4).
4. Call 911.

Additional Care

- Reassure the victim
- Monitor the ABCs until help arrives

Sucking Chest Wound

A sucking chest wound is an open wound in the chest caused by a penetrating injury. The wound lets air move in and out of the chest during breathing. This wound can be life threatening because breathing can be affected.

When You See

- Air moving in or out of a penetrating chest wound

Do This First

1. Put a thin sterile dressing over the wound.
2. Cover the dressing with a plastic bag or wrap to make an air-tight seal. As the victim exhales, tape it in place on three sides, leaving one side untaped to let exhaled air escape (Figure 6-5).
3. Position victim lying down inclined toward the injured side.
4. Call 911.

Additional Care

- If victim's breathing becomes more difficult, remove the plastic bandage to let air escape; then reapply it
- Monitor the ABCs until help arrives

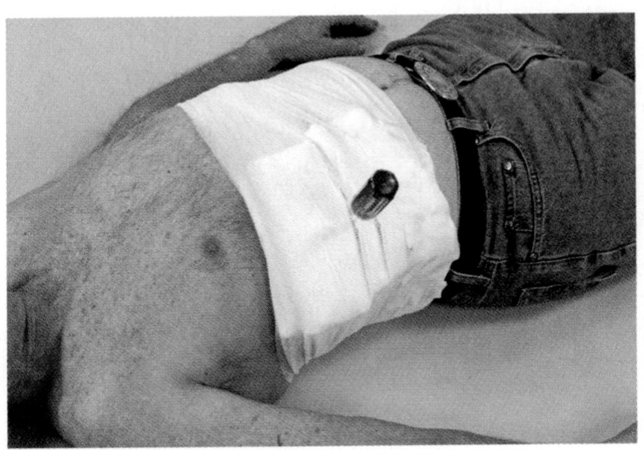

Figure 6-4 Bandage around an object impaled in the chest.

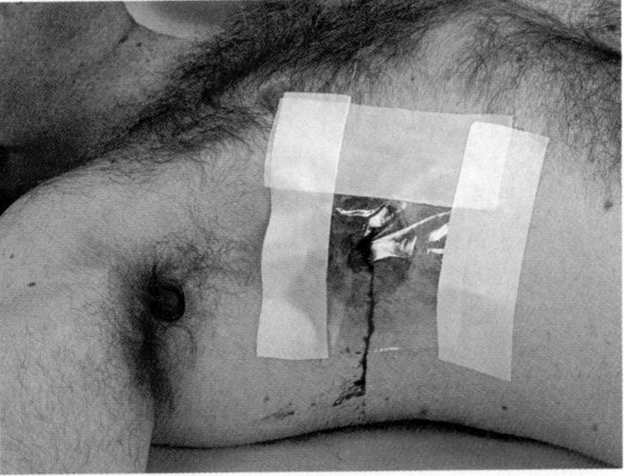

Figure 6-5 Tape only three sides to let air escape from a sucking chest wound.

Learning Checkpoint 2

1. True or False: Broken ribs are treated by taping the entire ribcage tightly.
2. Immobilize the arm of a victim with a rib fracture to
   a. Prevent movement
   b. Ease pain
   c. Help immobilize that side of the chest
   d. All of the above
3. What should you do with a screwdriver you see embedded in the chest of an unresponsive coworker after an explosion in the tool room?

   ____

4. A gunshot victim has a small bleeding hole in the right side of his chest. You open his shirt to treat the bleeding and see air bubbles forming in the hole as air escapes. How do you dress this wound?

   ____

Abdominal Injuries

Abdominal injuries include closed and open wounds that result from a blow to the abdomen or a fall. These may involve internal and/or external bleeding, and organs may protrude from the wound. The victim needs immediate medical care even if no significant injuries can be seen.

Closed Abdominal Injury

A closed abdominal injury can be life threatening because internal organs may have ruptured and there may be serious internal bleeding.

When You See

- Signs of severe pain, tenderness in area
- Bruising
- Swollen or rigid abdomen

Do This First

1. Carefully position the victim on his or her back and loosen any tight clothing. Allow the victim to bend knees slightly if this eases the pain.
2. Call 911.
3. Treat the victim for shock and monitor the ABCs.

Additional Care

- Continue to monitor the victim's ABCs until help arrives

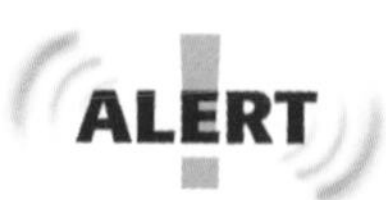

Abdominal Injury

Do not let the victim eat or drink.

Open Abdominal Wound

When You See

- Open abdominal wound
- Bleeding
- Organs possibly protruding from wound

Do This First

1. Lay the victim on his or her back and loosen any tight clothing. Allow the victim to bend knees slightly if this eases the pain.
2. If organs are protruding through the wound opening, do not try to push them back in. Cover the wound with a dressing moistened with sterile or clean water, or plastic wrap if water is unavailable.
3. Cover the moistened dressing with a large dry sterile dressing and tape it loosely in place.
4. Call 911.
5. Treat the victim for shock and monitor the ABCs (Figure 6-6).

Additional Care

- Monitor the victim's ABCs until help arrives

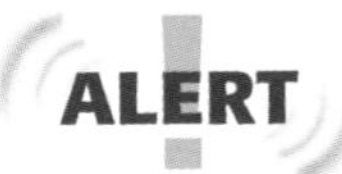

Open Abdominal Wound

Do not push protruding organs back inside the abdomen, but keep them from drying out with a moist dressing or plastic covering.

Learning Checkpoint 3

1. After an emergency at a construction site you find an unresponsive victim on the ground, his shirt torn open. Which of the following are signs and symptoms he may have a closed abdominal injury? (Check all that apply.)

   _____ Bruises below the ribcage _____ Pupils of eyes look small

   _____ Noisy breathing _____ Swollen abdomen

   _____ Skin feels hot all over _____ Skin around navel feels rigid

2. Describe the best position to put a victim in with either an open or closed abdominal wound.

   ____

3. True or False: To treat a victim for shock, help maintain normal body temperature.
4. If the victim has an organ protruding from an open abdominal wound, what should you do?
   - a. Push the organ back into the abdomen
   - b. Put a clean, dry dressing over the wound
   - c. Leave the wound exposed to the air
   - d. Cover the wound with a moist dressing or plastic wrap
5. In what circumstances do you call 911 for a victim with an open or closed abdominal wound?

   ____

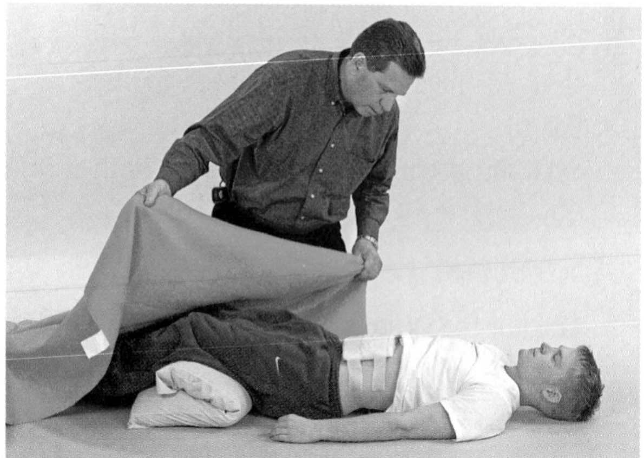

Figure 6-6 After dressing the abdominal wound, treat for shock while waiting for help.

Do This First

1. Help the victim lie on his or her back and bend knees slightly if this eases the pain.
2. Immobilize the victim's legs by padding between the legs and then bandaging them together, unless this causes more pain (Figure 6-7).
3. Call 911.
4. Treat the victim for shock and monitor the ABCs.

Additional Care

- Monitor the victim's ABCs until help arrives

Pelvic Injuries

A broken pelvis may cause severe internal bleeding and organ damage. A broken pelvis can be a life-threatening injury for some victims such as the elderly.

When You See

- Signs of pain and tenderness around the hips
- Inability to walk or stand
- Signs and symptoms of shock

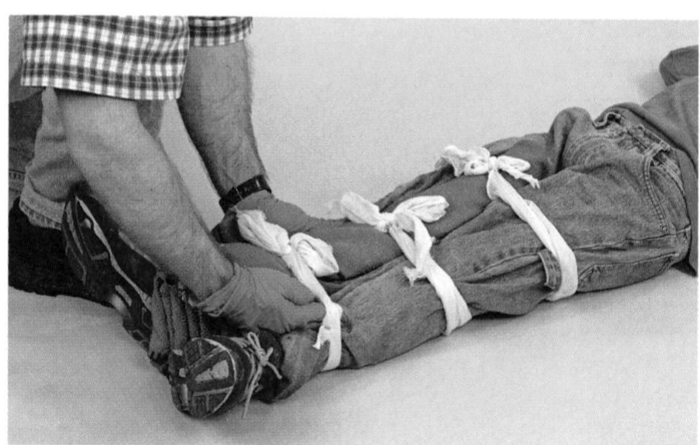

Figure 6-7 Bandage legs together for pelvic injury.

Learning Checkpoint 4

1. First aid for a pelvic fracture prevents __________ of the area.
2. True or False: Internal bleeding can be severe with a broken pelvis.
3. True or False: Bending the victim's knees slightly may ease the pain of a broken pelvis.

Chapter

7 Bone, Joint, and Muscle Injuries

CHAPTER PREVIEW

- Fractures
- Joint Injuries
- Muscle Injuries
- RICE
- Splinting the Extremities

Injuries of the bones, joints, and muscles are among the most common injuries both at work and in the home. Fractures are generally the most serious, although dislocations and sprains can also be very serious. Fortunately, most musculoskeletal injuries do not involve fractures or dislocations (Figure 7-1).

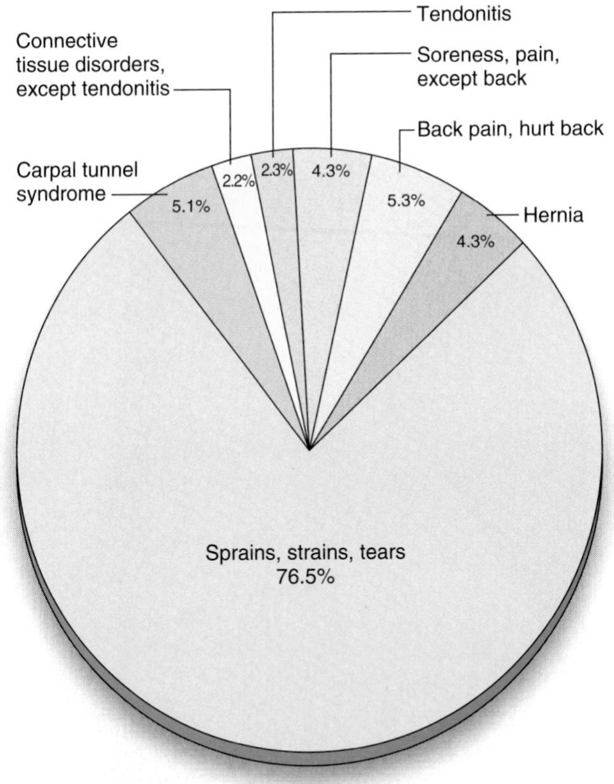

Figure 7-1 Musculoskeletal disorders causing days away from work by nature of injury or illness. *Source:* U.S. Department of Labor, Bureau of Labor Statistics. Survey of Occupational Injuries and Illnesses, 2001.

FRACTURES

A **fracture** is a broken bone. The bone may be completely broken with the pieces separated, or it may be only cracked. With a **closed fracture** the skin is not broken. With an **open fracture** there is an open wound at the fracture site, and bone may protrude through the wound (Figure 7-2). Bleeding can be severe with fractures of large bones, and organs nearby may also be injured.

When You See

- A deformed body part (compare to other side of body) (Figure 7-3)
- Signs of pain
- Swelling, discoloration of skin
- Inability to use the body part
- Bone exposed in a wound
- Victim heard or felt a bone snap
- Possible signs and symptoms of shock

Do This First

1. Have the victim rest and immobilize the area. With an extremity, also immobilize the joints above and below the fracture.
2. Call 911 for a large bone fracture. A victim with a fractured hand or foot may be transported to the emergency room.
3. With an open fracture, cover the wound with a dressing and apply gentle pressure around the fracture area only if needed to control bleeding.
4. Put ice or a cold pack on the area.

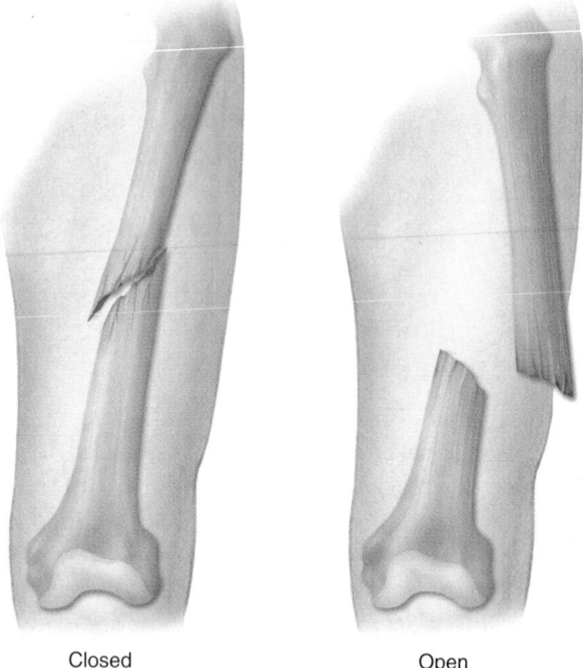

Figure 7-2 Closed and open fractures.

5. If help may be delayed or if the victim is to be transported, use a splint to keep the area immobilized (see later section on splints). Elevate a splinted arm.

Additional Care

- Treat the victim for shock
- Monitor the victim's ABCs
- Remove clothing and jewelry if they may cut off circulation as swelling occurs

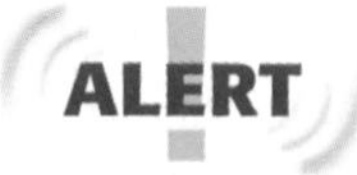

Fracture

Do not try to align the ends of a broken bone.
Do not give the victim anything to eat or drink.

Joint Injuries

Injuries to joints include dislocations and sprains. In a **dislocation,** one or more bones have been moved out of the normal position in a joint. A **sprain** is an injury to ligaments and other structures in a joint. Both kinds of joint injuries often look similar to a fracture.

Dislocations

It is not always possible to tell a dislocation from a closed fracture, but the first aid is very similar.

When You See

- The joint is deformed (compare to other side of body)
- Signs of pain
- Swelling
- Inability to use the body part

Do This First

1. Have the victim rest and immobilize the area in the position in which you find it (Figure 7-4).
2. Call 911. A victim with a dislocated bone in the hand or foot may be transported to the emergency room.

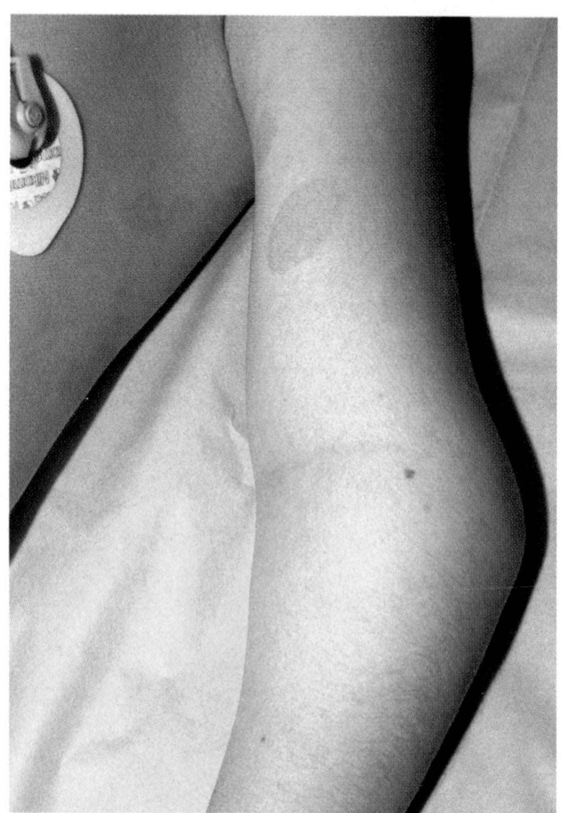

Figure 7-3 An obvious deformity may indicate a fracture.

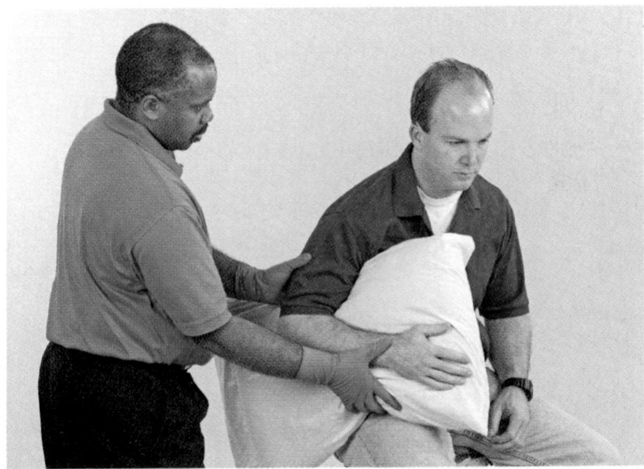

Figure 7-4 Immobilize and support a dislocated shoulder.

3. Put ice or a cold pack on the area.
4. If help may be delayed or if the victim is to be transported, use a splint to keep the area immobilized (see later section on splints).

Additional Care

- Treat the victim for shock
- Monitor the victim's ABCs
- Remove clothing and jewelry if they may cut off circulation as swelling occurs

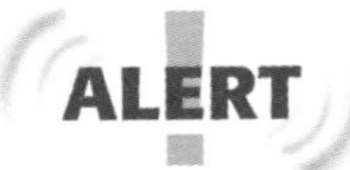

Dislocation

Do not try to put the displaced bone back in place. Do not let the victim eat or drink.

Sprains

Sprains can range from mild to severe. It may be difficult to tell a severe sprain from a fracture, but the first aid is similar for both. The ankles, knees, wrists, and fingers are the body parts most often sprained.

When You See

- Signs of pain
- Swollen joint
- Bruising of joint area
- Inability to use joint

Do This First

1. Have the victim rest and immobilize the area in the position in which you find it.
2. Put ice or a cold pack on the area and then wrap joint with a compression bandage (Figure 7-5).
3. Use a soft splint (bandage, pillow, blanket) to immobilize and support the joint.
4. Elevate a sprained hand or ankle above the level of the heart (Figure 7-6).
5. Seek medical attention.

Additional Care

- Remove clothing or jewelry if they may cut off circulation as swelling occurs

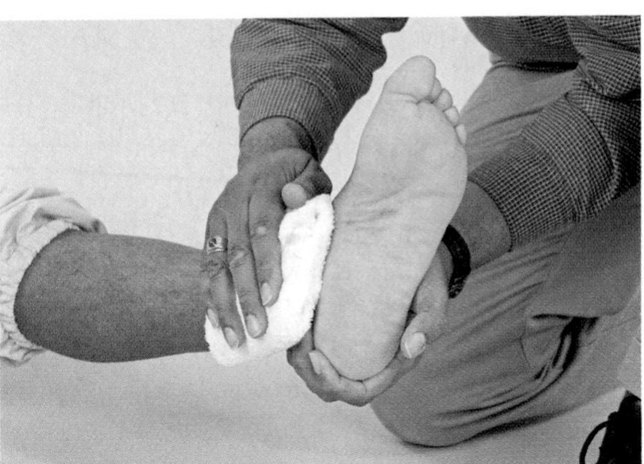

Figure 7-5 Put ice or a cold pack on the area.

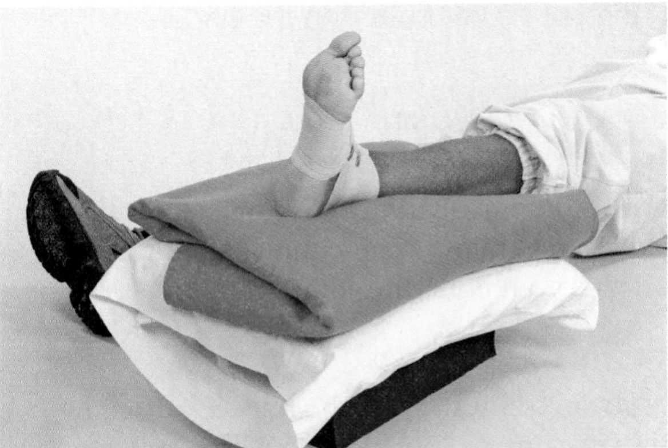

Figure 7-6 Put a compression bandage on a sprain and elevate.

Learning Checkpoint 1

1. True or False: Call 911 for a fracture of a large bone such as the thigh bone.

2. When immobilizing a fracture injury, what body area should be immobilized?

a. The immediate fracture area

b. The fracture area and the joint above it

c. The fracture area and both the joints above and below it

d. The entire victim

3. True or False: With a fracture, you may also need to treat the victim for shock.

4. The signs and symptoms of a bone or joint injury include which of the following? (Check all that apply.)

_____ Deformed area	_____ Pain
_____ Small or unequal pupils	_____ Inability to use part
_____ Skin is hot and red	_____ Fever
_____ Swelling	_____ Spasms and jerking of nearby muscles

5. True or False: A victim with a sprained ankle should "walk it off."

REMOVING A RING

When an injury to the hand or fingers causes swelling, the victim's watch or rings can cut off circulation. Try to remove a watch and rings before swelling occurs. Removal of a ring is easier if you first soak the finger in cold water or wrap it in a cold pack and then put oil or butter on the finger.

Muscle Injuries

Common muscle injuries include strains, contusions, and cramps. These injuries are usually less serious than bone and joint injuries.

Strains

A **strain** is a tearing of the muscle caused by overexerting or "pulling" a muscle. Back strains are common occupational injuries.

When You See

- Signs of dull or sharp pain when muscle is used
- Stiffness of the area
- Weakness or inability to use the muscle normally

Do This First

1. Rest the muscle.
2. Put ice or a cold pack on the area: 30 minutes on, then at least 30 minutes off.
3. With an extremity, wrap a compression bandage around the muscle.
4. Elevate the limb.

Additional Care

- Seek medical attention if pain is severe or persists

Contusions

A **contusion** is a bruised muscle as may result from a blow.

When You See

- Signs of pain
- Swollen, tender area
- Skin discoloration (black and blue)

Do This First

1. Rest the muscle.
2. Put ice or a cold pack on the area: 30 minutes on, then at least 30 minutes off.
3. With an extremity, wrap a compression bandage around the muscle.
4. Elevate the limb.

Additional Care

- Seek medical attention if pain is severe or persists

Cramps

A **muscle cramp** is a tightening of a muscle usually because of prolonged use. Cramps are common in the legs, stomach, back, or any muscle that is overused. These cramps are different from heat cramps, which result from fluid loss in hot environments (see Chapter 10).

When You See

- Signs of muscle pain and tightness

Do This First

1. Gently stretch out the muscle if possible.
2. Massage the muscle.

Additional Care

- Drink plenty of fluids

RICE

The RICE acronym is an easy way to remember how to treat all bone, joint, and muscle injuries. With this procedure you do not have to know whether the injury is a fracture, dislocation, sprain, or strain as they are treated in the same manner.

R = Rest
I = Ice
C = Compression
E = Elevation

Rest

Any movement of a musculoskeletal injury can cause further injury, pain, and swelling. Have the victim rest until medical help arrives. Rest is also important for healing.

Learning Checkpoint 2

1. True or False: For a muscle strain, keep an ice pack on the injury for at least 2 hours.
2. True or False: Vigorous massage is the best treatment for a muscle contusion.
3. True or False: You can tell a contusion from a fracture because only a contusion causes an area of skin discoloration.
4. Name two things you can do to ease a muscle cramp.

____

Perform the Skill

RICE Procedure for a Wrist Injury

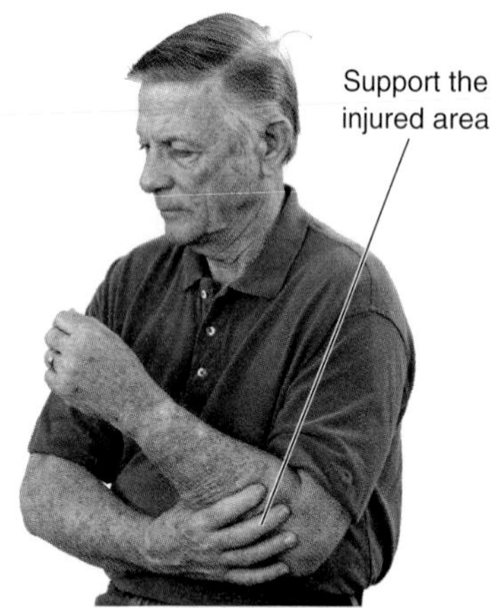
Support the injured area

1 Rest the injured wrist.

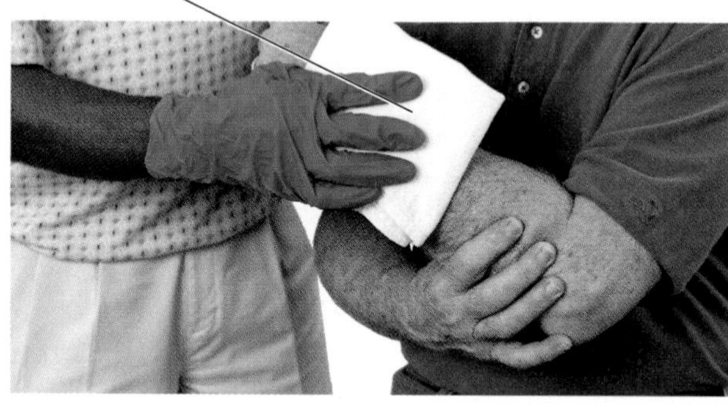
Apply cold for 30 minutes at a time

2 Put ice or cold pack on the injured area.

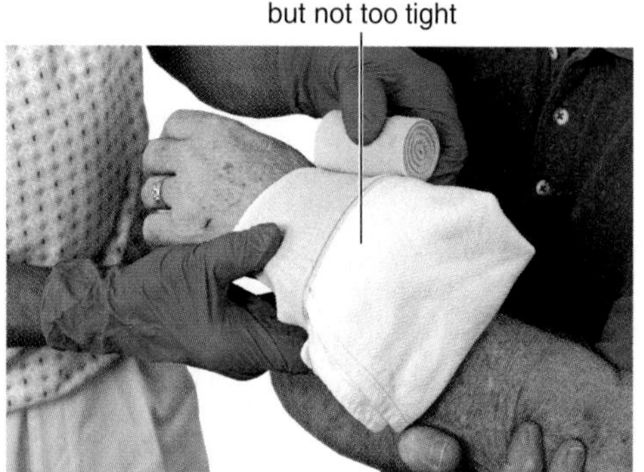
Bandage snuggly but not too tight

3 Compress the injured area with an elastic roller bandage.

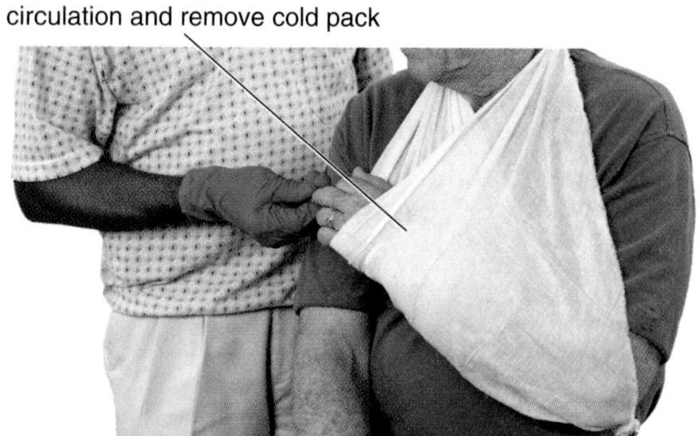
Remember to check circulation and remove cold pack

4 Elevate the injured area. Use a sling to hold the wrist in place.

Ice

Cold reduces swelling, lessens pain, and minimizes bruising. Put ice or a cold pack on the injury (except for an open fracture) as soon as possible. Cubed or crushed ice in a plastic bag, or an improvised cold pack such as a bag of frozen peas or a cloth pad soaked in cold water, can be applied directly on the injured area. A commercial cold pack should be wrapped in cloth to prevent direct skin contact because it may be cold enough to freeze the skin.

Cold works best if applied to the injury as soon as possible, preferably within 10 minutes. Apply it 30 minutes on and 30 minutes off for the first few hours, then for 20 to 30 minutes at a time every 2 or 3 hours for the first 24 to 48 hours, or for 72 hours for severe injuries.

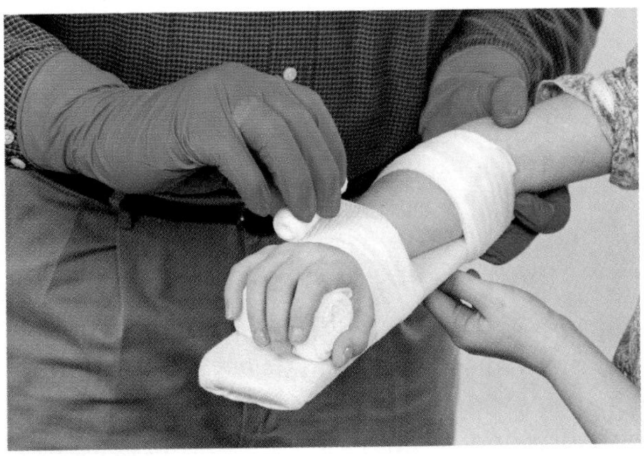
(a) Rigid splint.

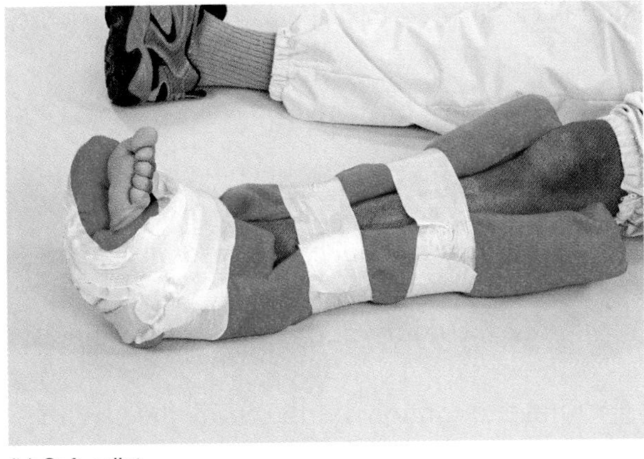
(b) Soft splint.

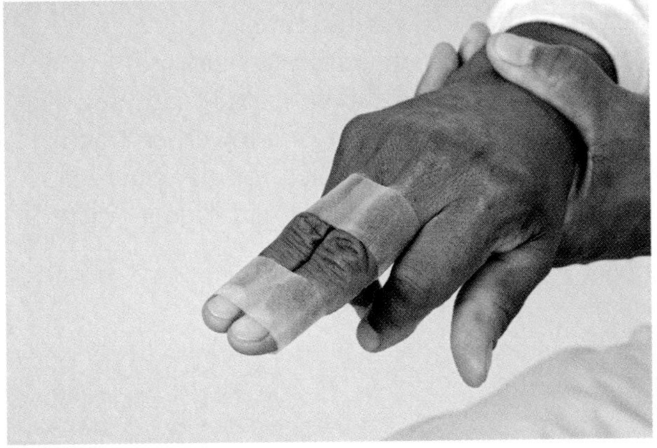
(c) Anatomic splint.

Figure 7-7 Examples of splints.

Compression

Compression of an injured extremity is done with an elastic roller bandage. Compression helps prevent internal bleeding and swelling. Wrap the bandage over the injured area. It also can be used around a cold pack. Check the fingers or toes frequently to make sure circulation is not cut off.

Elevation

Elevating an injured arm or leg also helps prevent swelling and control internal or external bleeding. Splint a fracture first, and elevate it only if moving the limb does not cause pain.

Splinting the Extremities

When a victim has a fracture, dislocation, or sprain in an arm or leg, the arm or leg may be splinted if the victim is at risk for moving the injured area unless help is expected within a few minutes. Always splint an extremity before transporting the victim to a healthcare provider or emergency room. Splinting helps prevent further injury, reduces pain, and minimizes bleeding and swelling.

Types of Splints

Splints can be made from many different materials at hand. There are three types of splints (**Figure 7-7**):

- **Rigid splints** may be made from a board, a piece of plastic or metal, a rolled newspaper or magazine, or thick cardboard.
- **Soft splints** may be made from a pillow, folded blanket or towel, or a triangular bandage folded into a sling.
- **Anatomic splints** involve splinting an injured leg to the uninjured leg or splinting fingers together.

Splints can be tied in place with bandages, belts, neckties, or strips of cloth torn from clothing.

Guidelines for Splinting

- Put a dressing on any open wound before splinting the area
- Splint only if it does not cause more pain for the victim
- Splint the injury in the position you find it (**Figure 7-8**)
- Splint to immobilize the entire area. With an extremity, splint the joints above and below the injured area.
- Put padding such as cloth between the splint and the victim's skin
- Put splints on both sides of a fractured bone if possible
- Elevate the splinted extremity if possible
- Apply ice or a cold pack to the injury around the splint
- With a splinted extremity, check the fingers or toes frequently to make sure circulation is not cut off. Swelling, bluish discoloration, tingling or numbness, and cold skin are signs and symptoms of reduced circulation. If any of these are noted, the splint should be removed.

Follow the steps shown in the following skill examples to splint an arm or leg. After splinting an arm, secure with a sling and binder. A sling supports and elevates an injury of the hand or forearm. A sling may also be used to minimize movement and support the area with a shoulder dislocation or rib fracture. A leg fracture can be splinted using either a rigid splint or an anatomic splint (as shown in the example). The example shows splinting of a lower leg fracture. A similar splint can be used for an upper leg fracture, with the bandages tied higher (including the hips).

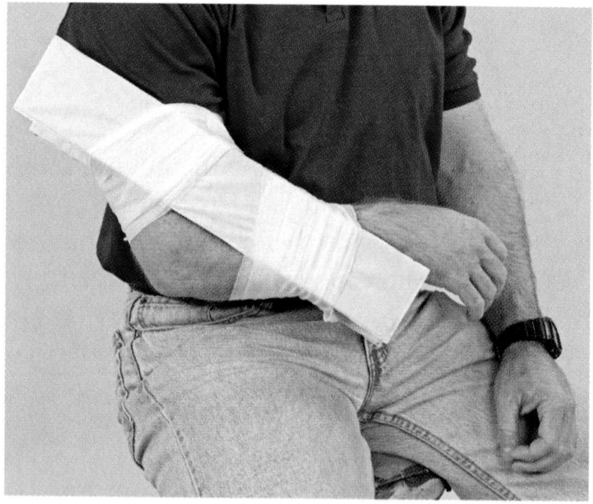

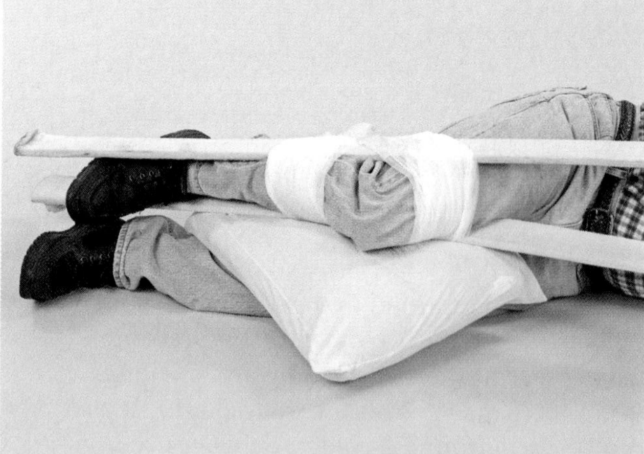

Figure 7-8 Splint an injury in the position found, such as this elbow fracture and knee injury. Do not try to straighten the limb to splint it.

Perform the Skill

Splinting an Arm

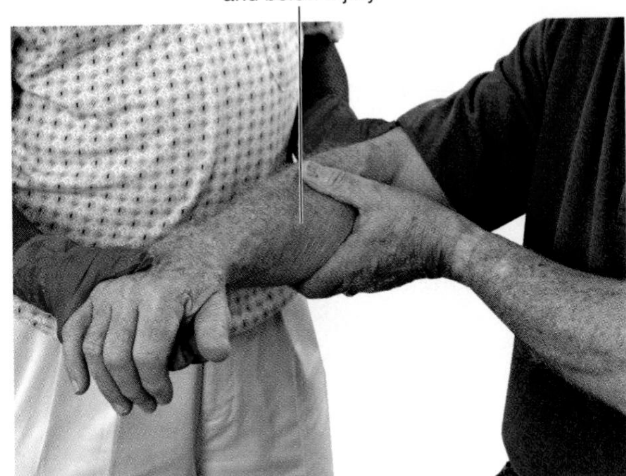
Support above
and below injury

1 Support the arm.

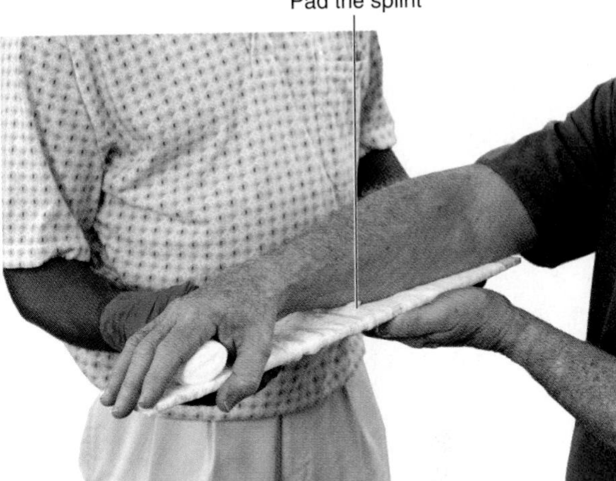
Pad the splint

2 Position the arm on a rigid splint.

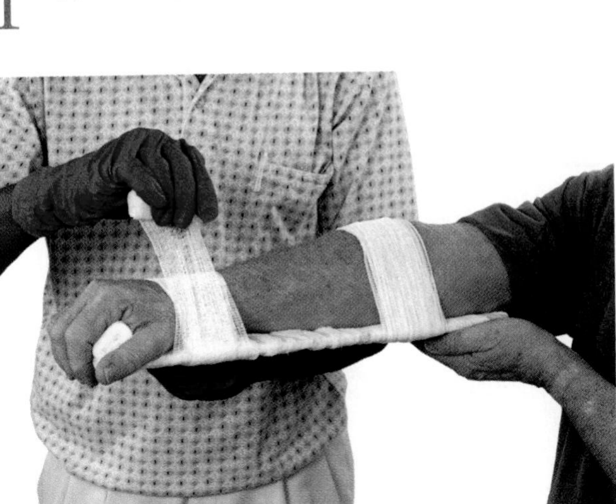

3 Secure the splint.

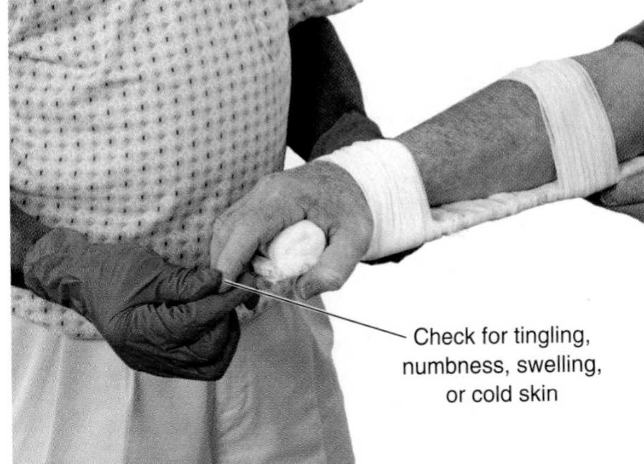
Check for tingling,
numbness, swelling,
or cold skin

4 Check circulation.

Perform the Skill

Making an Arm Sling and Binder

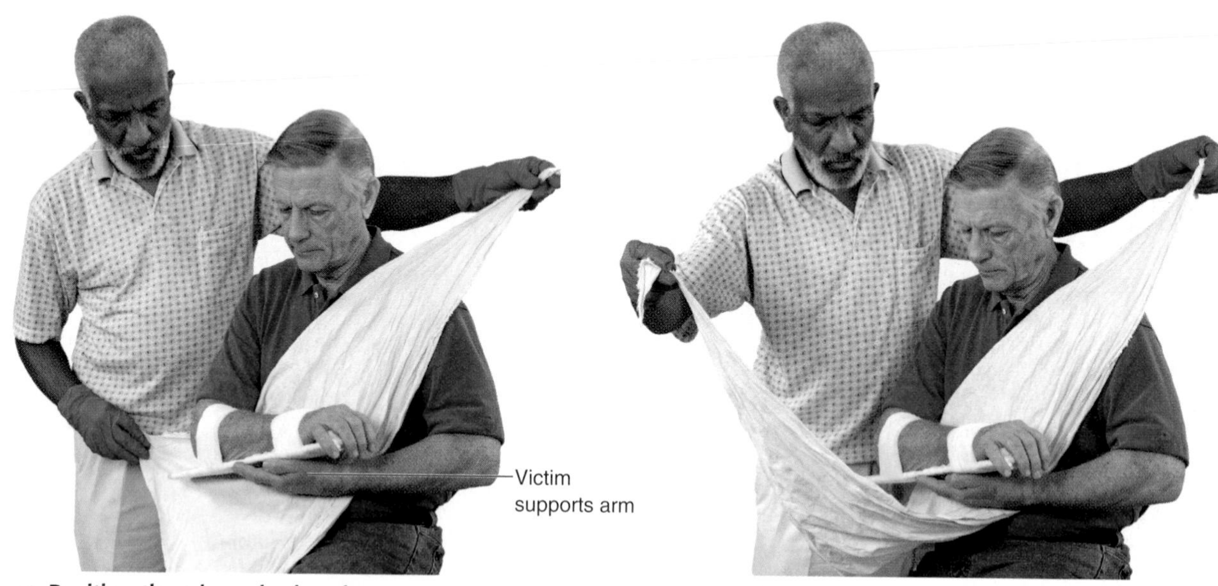
Victim
supports arm

1 Position the triangular bandage.

2 Bring up the lower end of the bandage to the opposite side of the neck.

3 Tie the ends.

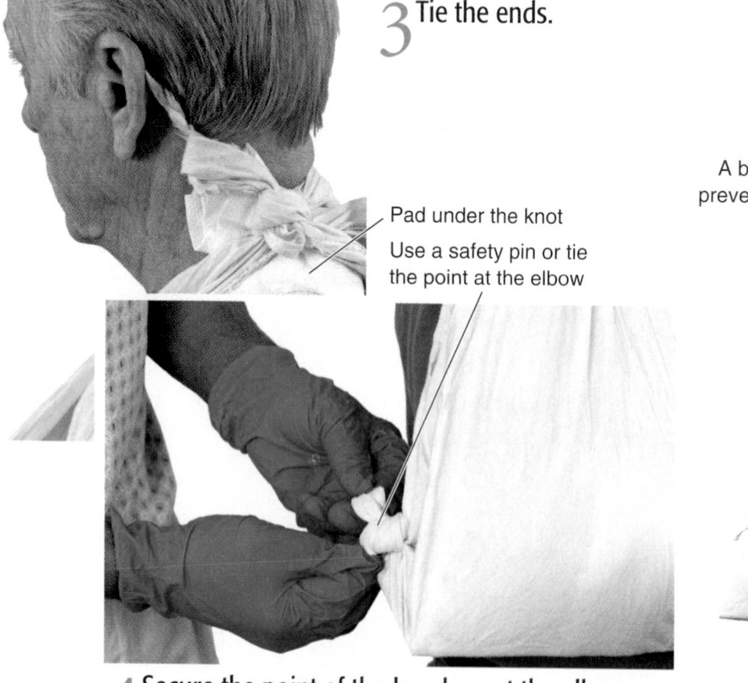
Pad under the knot
Use a safety pin or tie
the point at the elbow

4 Secure the point of the bandage at the elbow.

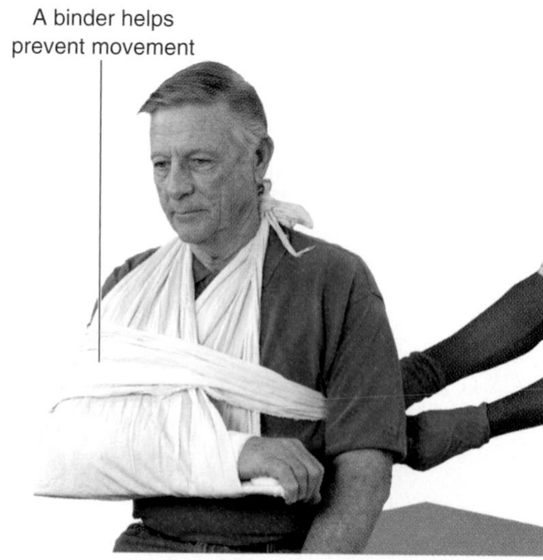
A binder helps
prevent movement

5 Tie a binder bandage over the sling and around the chest.

Perform the Skill

Splinting a Leg

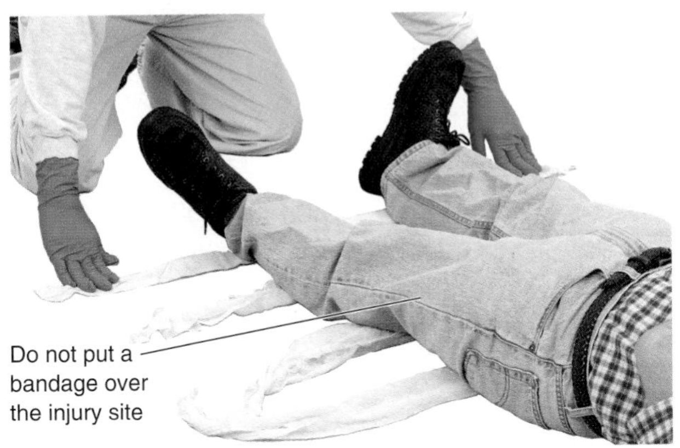
Do not put a
bandage over
the injury site

1 Gently slide 4 or 5 bandages or strips of cloth under both legs.

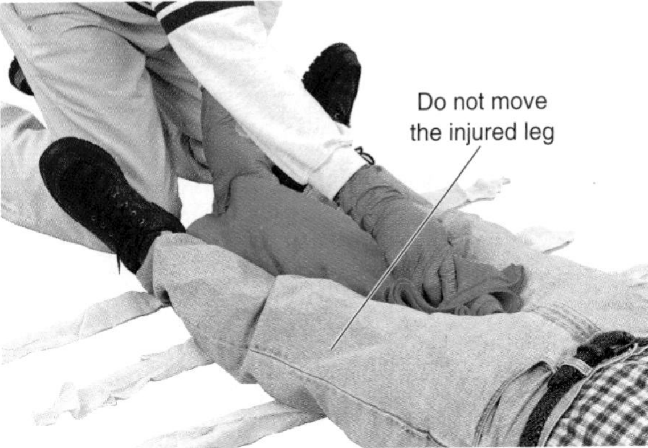
Do not move
the injured leg

2 Put padding between the legs.

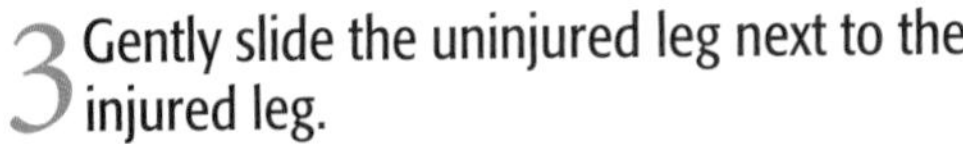

3 Gently slide the uninjured leg next to the injured leg.

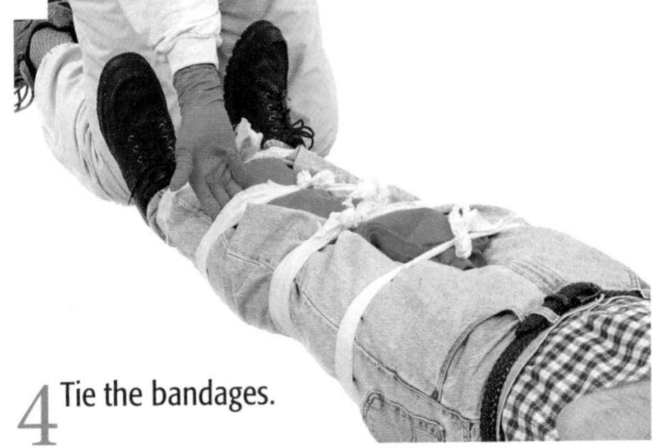

4 Tie the bandages.

Learning Checkpoint 3

1. Use RICE for:

a. Most musculoskeletal injuries

b. Fractures only

c. Muscle injuries only

d. Muscle and joint injuries only

2. True or False: Putting a cold pack directly on the skin is the best way to relieve pain and reduce swelling.

3. What is important about how you apply a compression bandage?

a. Use elastic roller bandage

b. Put the cold pack under the bandage, when needed

c. Check that circulation is not cut off

d. All of the above

4. Describe the steps you would follow to use RICE for a fractured or sprained ankle.

____

5. You encounter a victim with an obviously fractured forearm. What materials might you be able to find in your own work site that you can use to make a rigid splint?

____

6. When using a splint, which of the following are actions you should take? (Check all that apply.)

_____ Put a heating pad on the area

_____ Straighten out a limb before splinting it

_____ Dress an open wound before splinting

_____ Pad the splint

_____ Put a cold pack around splint

_____ Splint in position found

7. You are called to the scene where a coworker is lying on the ground with obvious severe pain in one leg after a piece of equipment fell on it. You cannot tell whether the bone is broken, but there is no open wound and the victim says it really hurts to move the leg. What should you do?

____

Chapter 8 Sudden Illness

CHAPTER PREVIEW

- Heart Attack
- Angina
- Stroke
- Respiratory Distress
- Fainting
- Seizures
- Severe Abdominal Pain
- Diabetic Emergencies

Many different illnesses may occur suddenly and become medical emergencies. You do not have to know for sure what the victim's specific illness is before you give first aid.

General signs and symptoms of sudden illness:

- Person feels ill, dizzy, confused, or weak
- Skin color changes (flushed or pale), sweating
- Nausea, vomiting

General care for sudden illness:

1. Call 911 for unexplained sudden illness.
2. Help victim rest and avoid getting chilled or overheated.
3. Reassure the victim.
4. Do not give the victim anything to eat or drink.
5. Monitor the ABCs and give care as needed.

Heart Attack

Heart attack is a sudden reduced blood flow to the heart muscle. It is a medical emergency because it can lead to cardiac arrest. Heart attack can occur at any age. The signs and symptoms of heart attack vary considerably, from vague chest discomfort (which the victim may confuse with heartburn) to crushing pain, with or without other symptoms. The victim may have no signs and symptoms at all before collapsing suddenly. Often the victim has milder symptoms that come and go for two or three days before the heart attack occurs. It is important to consider the possibility of heart attack with a wide range of symptoms rather than expecting a clearly defined situation (Figure 8-1).

FACTS ABOUT HEART ATTACK

- Half a million people a year in the U.S. die from heart attacks—many of whom could have been saved by prompt first aid and medical treatment.

- Heart attack results from coronary artery disease, which can often be prevented or minimized with a healthy diet, exercise, not smoking, and regular medical care.
- Heart attack is more likely in those with a family history of heart attacks.
- One-fifth of heart attack victims do not have chest pain—but often have other symptoms.
- Heart attack victims typically deny that they're having a heart attack. Do not let them talk you out of getting help!

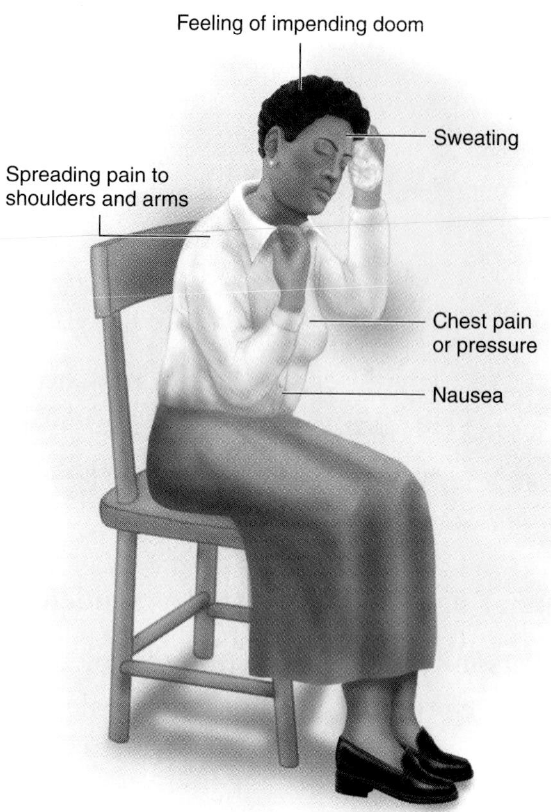

Figure 8-1 Signs and symptoms of a heart attack.

When You See

- Complaints of persistent pressure, tightness, ache, or pain in the chest
- Pain may spread to neck, shoulders, or arms
- Shortness of breath
- Dizziness, lightheadedness, feeling of impending doom
- Pale skin, sweating
- Nausea

Do This First

1. Call 911 immediately, even if the victim says it is not serious.
2. Help the victim rest in a comfortable position. Loosen constricting clothing.
3. Allow the victim to take one aspirin (unless allergic).
4. Stay with the victim, and be reassuring and calming.

Additional Care

- Ask the victim if he or she is taking heart medication, and help obtain the medication
- Do not let the victim eat or drink anything
- Monitor the ABCs and give care as needed

Angina

Angina is a chest pain caused by heart disease that usually happens after intense activity or exertion. The pain usually lasts only a few minutes. People usually know when they have angina and may carry medication for it.

Help a person with angina take his or her own medication and rest. If the pain persists more than 10 minutes or stops and then returns, or if the victim has other heart attack symptoms, give first aid as for a heart attack.

Stroke

A stroke, also called a brain attack, is an interruption of blood flow to a part of the brain, killing nerve cells and affecting the victim's functioning. A stroke victim needs medical help immediately to decrease the chance of permanent damage. Strokes are more common in older adults. Over 500,000 Americans have strokes every year.

When You See

- Sudden, severe headache
- Sudden weakness or numbness of face, arm, or leg on one side
- Dizziness, confusion, difficulty understanding speech
- Difficulty speaking or swallowing, vision problems
- Changing levels of responsiveness or unresponsiveness

Do This First

1. Call 911.
2. Monitor the ABCs and give care as needed.
3. Have the victim lie on his or her back with head and shoulders slightly raised. Loosen a constrictive collar.
4. If necessary, turn the victim's head to the side to allow drool or vomit to drain (Figure 8-2).

Additional Care

- Keep the victim warm and quiet until help arrives
- Put an unresponsive victim in the recovery position

Learning Checkpoint 1

1. True or False: With an unknown sudden illness, do not give the victim anything to eat or drink.

2. Check off the common signs and symptoms of heart attack:

_____ **a.** Skin red and flushed
_____ **b.** Tingling in fingers and toes
_____ **c.** Shortness of breath
_____ **d.** Chest pain or pressure
_____ **e.** Sweating
_____ **f.** Nausea
_____ **g.** Headache
_____ **h.** Pale skin
_____ **i.** Unusual cheerfulness
_____ **j.** Dizziness

3. How do you decide if a victim's chest pain may be a heart attack or angina?

____

4. The immediate first action to take for a heart attack victim is ___________.

5. It may be important to position a stroke victim such that:

a. Fluids drain from the mouth

b. The victim's head is protected from injury during convulsions

c. The victim can sit up even if partially paralyzed

d. The victim's head is lower than rest of the body

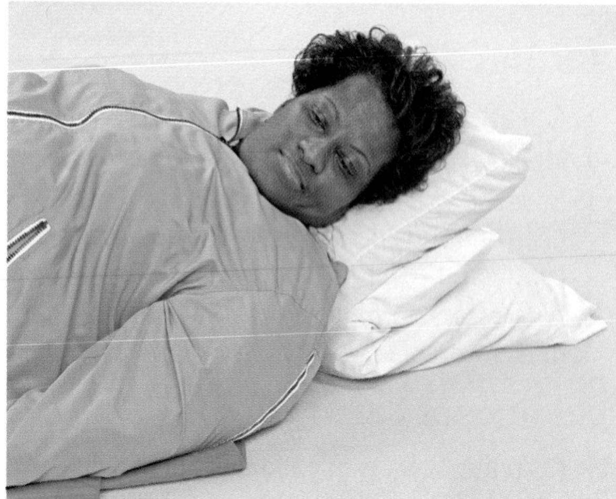

Figure 8-2 Position a victim who has had a stroke.

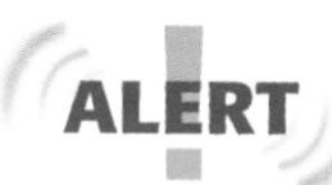

Stroke

Do not let a stroke victim eat or drink anything.

Respiratory Distress

Respiratory distress, or difficulty breathing, can be caused by many different illnesses and injuries. If you can know the cause of a victim's breathing difficulty, give first aid for that problem. Otherwise, give the general breathing care described below.

When You See

- Victim is gasping or unable to catch his or her breath
- Breathing is faster or slower, or deeper or shallower, than normal
- Breathing involves sounds such as wheezing or gurgling
- Victim feels dizzy or lightheaded

Do This First

1. Call 911 for sudden unexplained breathing problems.
2. Help the victim rest in position of easiest breathing.
3. Ask victim about any prescribed medicine he or she may have, and help the victim take it if needed.
4. Monitor the ABCs and give care as needed.

Additional Care

- Calm and reassure the victim (anxiety increases breathing distress)

Asthma

Asthma is a common problem affecting 1 in 20 adults and 1 in 7 children. In an asthma attack the airway becomes narrow and the person has difficulty breathing. Many asthma victims know they have the condition and carry medication for emergency situations (Figure 8-3). Untreated, a severe asthma attack can be fatal.

When You See

- Wheezing and difficulty breathing and speaking
- Dry, persistent cough
- Fear, anxiety
- Gray-blue skin
- Changing levels of responsiveness

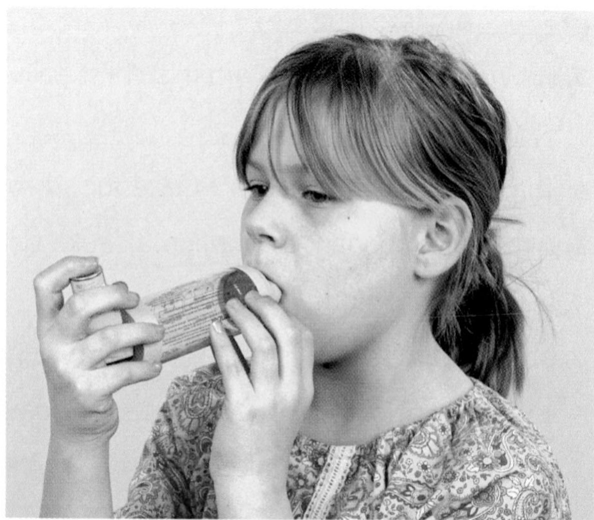

Figure 8-3 Many people with asthma use an inhaler.

Do This First

1. If the victim does not know he or she has asthma (first attack), call 911 immediately.
2. Help the victim use his or her medication (usually in an inhaler).
3. Help the victim rest and sit in a position for easiest breathing.
4. The victim may use the inhaler again in 5–10 minutes if needed.

Additional Care

- If the breathing difficulty persists after using the inhaler, call 911

Hyperventilation

Hyperventilation is fast, deep breathing caused by anxiety or stress.

When You See

- Very fast breathing rate
- Dizziness, faintness
- Tingling or numbness in hands and feet
- Muscle twitching or cramping

Do This First

1. Make sure there is no other cause for the breathing difficulty to care for.
2. Reassure the victim and ask him or her to try to breathe slowly.
3. Call 911 if the victim's breathing does not return to normal within a few minutes.

Additional Care

- A victim who often has this problem should seek medical care, because some medical conditions can cause rapid breathing

Learning Checkpoint 2

1. True or False: You cannot give first aid for a person with difficulty breathing unless you know the specific cause of the problem.
2. To help someone breathe easier:
   a. Position the victim flat on his or her back
   b. Have the victim stand, and clap him or her on the back with each breath
   c. Have the victim sit and put his or her head between the knees
   d. Let the victim find the position in which he or she can breathe most easily
3. What is the best thing a victim with asthma can do when having an asthma attack?

   ____
4. True or False: Have a hyperventilation victim breathe into a bag in order to start breathing normally again.
5. When should you call 911 for a victim who seems to be hyperventilating?

   ____

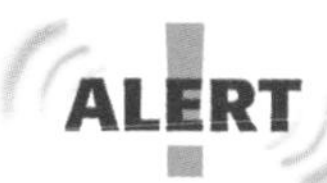

Hyperventilation

Do not ask the victim to breathe into a bag or other container. A victim who repeatedly rebreathes his or her exhaled air will not be getting enough oxygen.

Fainting

Fainting is caused by a temporary reduced blood flow to the brain. This commonly occurs in hot weather or after a prolonged period of inactivity, or from other causes such as fright or lack of food.

When You See

- Sudden brief loss of responsiveness and collapse
- Pale, cool skin, sweating

Do This First

1. Check the victim's ABCs and give care as needed.
2. Lay the victim down and raise the legs about 12 inches. Loosen constricting clothing.
3. Check for possible injuries caused by falling.
4. Reassure the victim as he or she recovers.

Additional Care

- Call 911 if the victim does not regain responsiveness soon or faints repeatedly
- Place an unresponsive victim in the recovery position to let the mouth drain in case of vomiting

Seizures

Seizures, or convulsions, result from a brain disturbance caused by many different conditions, including epilepsy, high fever in young children, certain injuries, electric shock, and other causes.

When You See

- *Minor seizures:* staring blankly ahead; slight twitching of lips, head, or arms and legs; other movements such as lip-smacking or chewing
- *Major seizures:* crying out and then becoming unresponsive; body becomes rigid and then shakes in convulsions; jaw may clench
- *Fever convulsions in young children:* hot, flushed skin; violent muscle twitching; arched back; clenched fists

Do This First

1. Prevent injury during the seizure by moving away dangerous objects and putting something flat and soft under the head (Figure 8-4).
2. Loosen clothing around the neck to ease breathing.
3. Gently turn the victim onto one side to help keep the airway clear if vomiting occurs.
4. Be reassuring as the victim regains responsiveness.

Additional Care

- Call 911 if the seizure last more than 5 minutes, if the victim is not known to have epilepsy, if the victim recovers very slowly or has trouble breathing or has another seizure, if the victim is pregnant or is wearing another medical ID, or if the victim is injured
- For an infant or child with fever convulsions, sponge the body with lukewarm water to help cool the victim, and call 911

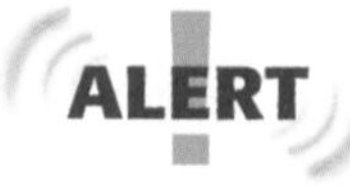

Seizure

Do not try to stop the victim's movements. Do not place any objects in the victim's mouth.

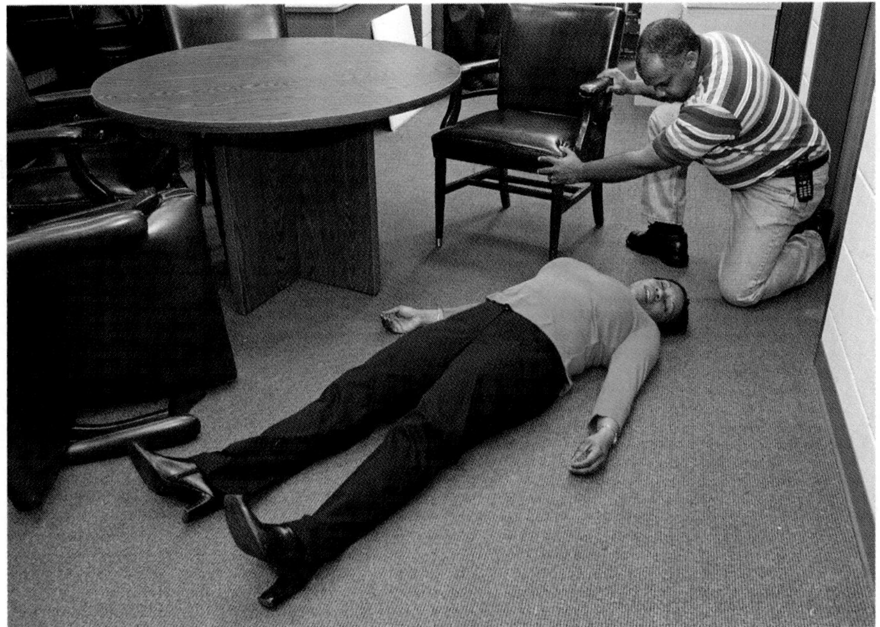

Figure 8-4 Protect a victim from injury during a seizure.

Severe Abdominal Pain

Abdominal injuries were described in Chapter 6; always call 911 for an abdominal injury. Abdominal pain may also result from illness ranging from minor conditions to serious medical emergencies. Urgent medical care is needed for any severe abdominal pain in these situations:

In adults:

- Sudden, severe, intolerable pain, or pain that causes awakening from sleep
- Pain that begins in general area of central abdomen and later moves to lower right
- Pain accompanied by fever, sweating, black or bloody stool, or blood in urine
- Pain in pregnancy or accompanying abnormal vaginal bleeding
- Pain accompanied by dry mouth, dizziness on standing, or decreased urination
- Pain accompanied by difficulty breathing
- Pain accompanied by vomiting blood or greenish-brown fluid

In young children:

- Pain that occurs suddenly, stops, and then returns without warning
- Pain accompanied by red or purple, jelly-like stool; or with blood or mucus in stool
- Pain accompanied by greenish-brown vomit
- Pain with swollen abdomen that feels hard
- Pain with a hard lump in lower abdomen or groin area

Diabetic Emergencies

People with diabetes sometimes have problems maintaining a balance of blood sugar and insulin in the body. Low blood sugar is called **hypoglycemia,** and high blood sugar is called **hyperglycemia.** Many factors can cause either of these conditions. Either can quickly progress to a medical emergency if the person is not treated. Diabetics often carry glucose tablets in case of low blood sugar (**Figure 8-5**).

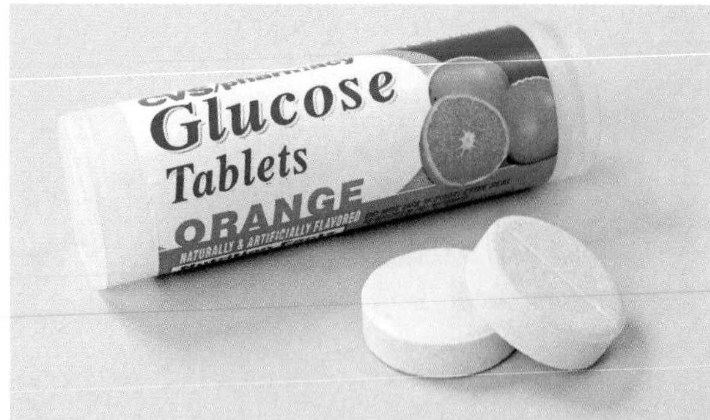

Figure 8-5 Diabetics often carry glucose tablets in case of low blood sugar.

Diabetic Emergency

If a diabetic victim becomes unresponsive, do not try to inject insulin or put food or fluids in the mouth.

Low Blood Sugar

When You See

- Sudden dizziness, shakiness, or mood change (even combativeness)
- Headache, confusion, difficulty paying attention
- Pale skin, sweating
- Hunger
- Clumsy, jerky movements
- Possible seizure

Do This First

1. Talk to the victim and confirm he or she has diabetes; look for a medical alert ID.
2. Give the victim sugar: 3 glucose tablets, ½ cup fruit juice, 1 or 2 sugar packets (but *not* non-sugar sweetener packets), or 5 to 6 pieces of hard candy (unless choking is a risk).
3. If the victim still feels ill or has signs and symptoms after 15 minutes, give more sugar.

Additional Care

- If victim becomes unresponsive or continues to have significant signs and symptoms, call 911 and monitor the victim's ABCs

High Blood Sugar

When You See

- Frequent urination
- Drowsiness
- Dry mouth, thirst
- Shortness of breath, deep rapid breathing
- Breath smells fruity
- Nausea, vomiting
- Eventual unresponsiveness

Do This First

1. Talk to the victim and confirm he or she has diabetes; look for a medical alert ID.
2. Have the victim follow his or her healthcare provider's instructions for hyperglycemia.
3. If you cannot judge whether the victim has low or high blood sugar, give sugar as for low blood sugar. If the victim does not improve in 15 minutes, seek medical care.
4. Call 911 if the victim becomes unresponsive or continues to have significant signs and symptoms.

Additional Care

- Put an unresponsive victim in the recovery position

Learning Checkpoint 3

1. When should you call 911 for a victim who faints?

____

2. True or False: When a person has fainted, lay him or her down and raise the head and shoulders about 12 inches.

3. For a victim having seizures:

a. Lay the victim face down on the floor

b. Ask others to help you hold the victim's head, arms, and legs still

c. Put something flat and soft under the victim's head

d. Put something wood, like a pencil, between the victim's teeth

4. Name at least three situations in which you should call 911 for a seizure victim.

____

5. What should you do for a young child whose abdomen is swollen and feels hard?

____

6. Check off common signs and symptoms of a low blood sugar diabetic emergency:

_____ **a.** Dizziness

_____ **b.** Hunger

_____ **c.** Rapid deep breathing

_____ **d.** Clumsiness

_____ **e.** Red, blotchy skin

_____ **f.** Sweating

_____ **g.** Confusion

_____ **h.** Swollen legs

7. In the late afternoon you come across a coworker who is acting oddly. She is sitting at her desk staring into space, and when you ask her if she is okay, she does not seem to understand what you are saying. She looks ill, her skin is pale, and she is sweating even though the room is not warm. Another employee comes over and tells you that this woman is diabetic and that he thinks she might have skipped lunch today. You cannot be sure whether she has low or high blood sugar. What should you do?

____

Chapter

9 Poisoning

CHAPTER PREVIEW

- Swallowed Poisons
- Inhaled Poisons
- Alcohol Abuse
- Drug Abuse or Overdose
- Poison Ivy, Oak, and Sumac
- Bites and Stings

SWALLOWED POISONS

Many substances in home and work settings are poisonous if swallowed.

When You See

- Open container of poisonous substance
- Nausea, vomiting, abdominal cramps
- Drowsiness, dizziness, disorientation
- Changing levels of responsiveness

Do This First

1. Determine what was swallowed, when, and how much.
2. *For a responsive victim,* call the national Poison Control Center (800-222-1222) immediately and follow their instructions.
3. *For an unresponsive victim,* check the ABCs, call 911, and provide care as needed.

Additional Care

- Put an unresponsive victim in the recovery position and be prepared for vomiting
- If a responsive victim's mouth or lips are burned by a corrosive chemical, rinse the mouth with cold water (without swallowing)

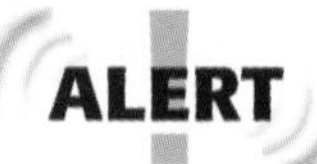

Swallowed Poison

Do not try to induce vomiting unless instructed by the Poison Control Center.

Food Poisoning

Food poisoning symptoms may begin soon after eating or within a day.

When You See

- Nausea and vomiting, signs of abdominal pain or cramps
- Diarrhea, possibly with blood
- Headache, fever

Do This First

1. Have the victim rest lying down.
2. Give the victim lots of fluids.
3. Seek medical attention.

Additional Care

- Check with others with whom victim has eaten recently

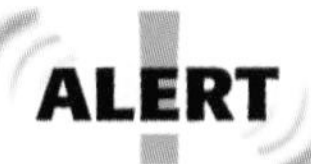

Botulism

Botulism is more likely from home-canned foods. If the victim experiences dizziness, muscle weakness, and difficulty talking or breathing, call 911.

PREVENTING FOOD POISONING

- Fully defrost frozen poultry and meat before cooking

- Fully cook poultry, meat, fish, and eggs to kill bacteria
- Do not keep cooked foods lukewarm a long time before serving

Wash hands before preparing food; wash anytime after touching uncooked poultry.

Inhaled Poisons

In work settings various gases and fumes may be present. Unless you know the specific treatment for inhaling a gas, care for a victim of suspected gas inhalation the same as for carbon monoxide.

Carbon Monoxide

Carbon monoxide is especially dangerous because it is invisible, odorless, and tasteless—and very lethal. Carbon monoxide may be present from motor vehicle exhaust, a faulty furnace, industrial equipment, or fire. Exposure to large amounts causes an immediate poisoning reaction; a slow or small leak may cause gradual poisoning with less dramatic symptoms. To prevent poisoning, carbon monoxide detectors should be used along with smoke detectors in appropriate locations.

When You See

- Headache
- Dizziness, lightheadedness, confusion, weakness
- Nausea, vomiting
- Signs of chest pain
- Convulsions
- Changing levels of responsiveness

Do This First

1. Immediately move the victim into fresh air.
2. Call 911 even if the victim starts to recover.
3. Monitor the ABCs and give care as needed.

Additional Care

- Put an unresponsive victim in the recovery position
- Loosen tight clothing around neck or chest

Alcohol Abuse

Excessive alcohol consumption causes problems that may lead to a medical emergency.

When You See

- Smell of alcohol about the person
- Flushed, moist face
- Slurred speech, staggering
- Changing levels of responsiveness

Do This First

1. Check for injuries or illness. Do not assume alcohol is the factor involved. Note that victims with uncontrolled diabetes may appear as if they are intoxicated.
2. *For a responsive intoxicated person:*
   a. Stay with the person and protect from injury (take away car keys).
   b. Do not let the person lie down on his or her back.
3. *For an unresponsive intoxicated person:*
   a. Position the person in the recovery position; be prepared for vomiting.
   b. Monitor the ABCs and give care as needed.
   c. Call 911 if the victim's breathing is irregular, if seizures occur, or if the victim cannot be roused (coma).

Additional Care

- In a cold environment an intoxicated person is likely to experience hypothermia. Give appropriate care (see Chapter 10).

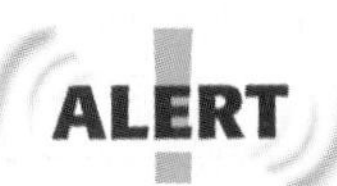

Intoxication

Intoxication makes some people hostile and violent. Stay a distance away and call police if violence threatens.

Drug Abuse or Overdose

A person under the influence of illegal drugs or having an overdose of a prescription medication may have a wide range of behaviors and symptoms, depending on the specific drug. Drug withdrawal can also be an emergency. In some cases it is impossible to know whether behavior or symptoms are caused by drugs or by an injury or sudden illness. Follow these general guidelines.

When You See

- Very small or large pupils of the eye
- Stumbling, clumsiness, drowsiness, incoherent speech
- Difficulty breathing (very slow or fast)
- Irrational or violent behavior
- Changing levels of responsiveness
- Evidence of a suicide attempt

Do This First

1. Put an unresponsive victim in the recovery position. Monitor the ABCs and give care as needed. Call 911.
2. For a responsive victim, first ensure it is safe to approach the person. If the person's behavior is erratic or violent, call 911 and stay a safe distance away.
3. Try to find out what drug the victim took. If there is evidence of an overdose, call 911.
4. If symptoms are minor and you know the substance taken, call the Poison Control Center and follow their instructions.

Additional Care

- Monitor the victim's condition while waiting for help
- Provide care for any condition that occurs (seizures, shock, cardiac arrest)

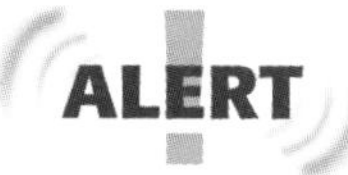

Drug Abuse

Do not try to reason with someone on drugs. The person may not act reasonably.

Learning Checkpoint 1

1. Check off the common signs and symptoms of a swallowed poison.

_____ **a.** Nausea
_____ **b.** Uncontrolled shaking
_____ **c.** Dizziness
_____ **d.** Drowsiness
_____ **e.** Red lips
_____ **f.** Vomiting
_____ **g.** Unresponsiveness
_____ **h.** Hyperactivity

2. Name one action you would take for a victim of food poisoning that you would ***not*** do for a victim of swallowed poison.

____

3. The first thing to do for a victim of carbon monoxide poisoning is:

a. Loosen tight clothing around the neck
b. Call 911
c. Move victim to fresh air
d. Position the victim in the recovery position

4. True or False: Alcohol intoxication may put the person at risk for injury but is never a medical emergency.

5. You see an intoxicated man lie down on his back and apparently pass out. What are the two most important actions to take?

____

6. True or False: You can tell when victims use an illegal drug because they always have dilated pupils.

7. Because of the way he is acting, you suspect a coworker is under the influence of a drug. In what situation would you call 911 for this person? When might you call the Poison Control Center instead?

____

8. You are called to the company lunchroom where an employee's visiting child is unresponsive on the floor. The cabinet under the sink is open, and the caps are off several bottles of cleaning products. Describe what actions you need to take.

____

Poison Ivy, Oak, and Sumac

Contact with these plants causes an allergic skin reaction in about half the population. Once the rash appears on the skin and has been washed, however, it cannot spread to other people; it is not a contagious condition but a reaction to a substance in the plant (**Figure 9-1**).

When You See

- Redness and extreme itching occur first
- Rash, blisters (may weep)
- Possible headache and fever

Do This First

1. Wash the area thoroughly with soap and water as soon as possible after contact.
2. For severe reactions or swelling on the face, the victim needs medical attention.
3. Treat itching with colloid oatmeal baths; a paste made of baking soda and water, calamine lotion, or topical hydrocortisone cream; and an oral antihistamine (Benadryl, for example).

Additional Care

- Wash clothing and shoes (and pets) that contacted the plants to prevent further spread

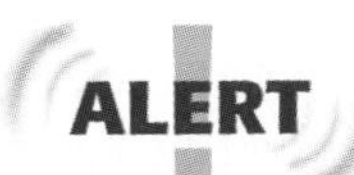

Poison Ivy/Oak/Sumac

Do not burn these poisonous plants to get rid of them as smoke also spreads the poisonous substance.

Bites and Stings

Animal Bites

Animal bites cause a wound and carry the risk of rabies, which can be fatal without prompt treatment. Rabies should be suspected in cases of unprovoked attacks, strangely acting animals, or wild (nondomestic) animals.

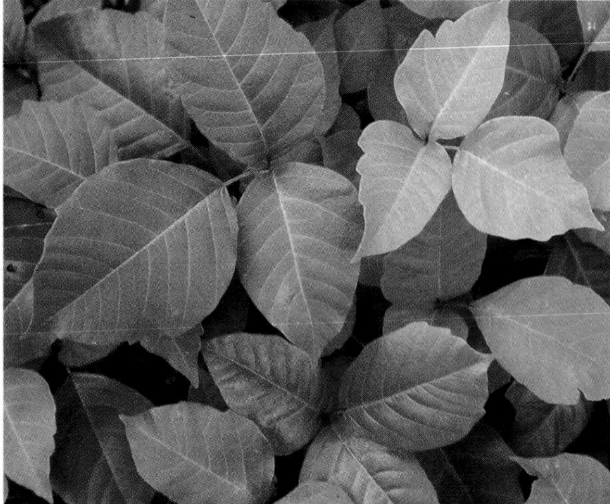

(a) Poison ivy

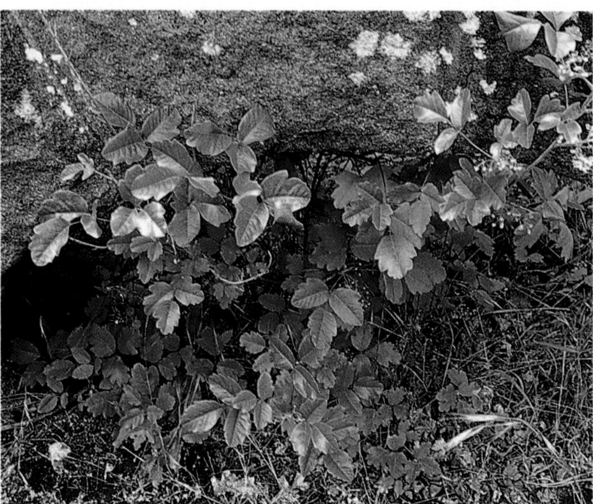

(b) Poison oak

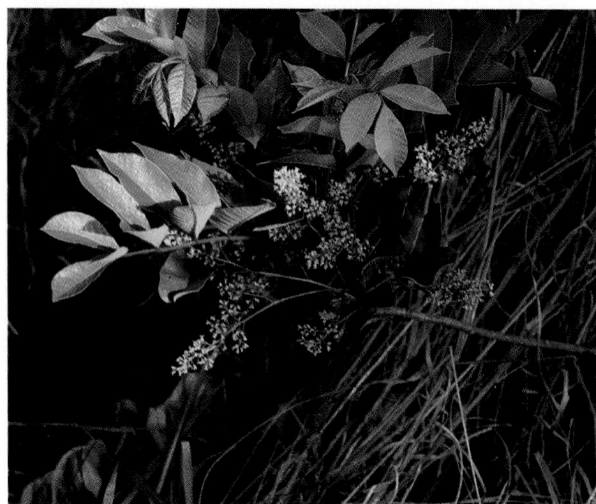

(c) Poison sumac

Figure 9-1 Common poisonous plants.

When You See

- Any animal bite

Do This First

1. Clean the wound with soap and water. Run water over the wound for 5 minutes (except when bleeding severely).
2. Control bleeding.
3. Cover the wound with a sterile dressing and bandage (see Chapter 3).
4. The victim should see a healthcare provider or go to the emergency room right away.

Additional Care

- Report all animal bites to local animal control officers or police. The law requires certain procedures to be followed when rabies is a risk.

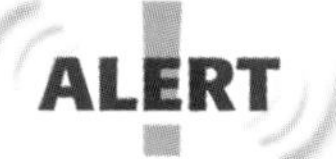

Animal Bite

Do not try to catch any animal that may have rabies.

Human Bites

Because our mouths are full of germs, a bite from a human can cause a wound infection.

When You See

- A human bite
- Open puncture wound
- Bleeding

Do This First

1. Clean the wound with soap and water. Run water over wound for 5 minutes (except when bleeding severely).
2. Control bleeding.
3. Cover the wound with a sterile dressing and bandage (see Chapter 3).

Learning Checkpoint 2

1. True or False: Never put water on a site of contact with poison ivy because of the risk of spreading the rash further.

2. When should a person with a poison ivy or oak rash see a healthcare provider?

____

3. Which of the following can help reduce the itching of poison ivy?

a. Hydrocortisone cream

b. Rubbing alcohol

c. A paste made with dishwasher detergent

d. All of the above

4. The victim should see a healthcare provider or go to the emergency room right away.

Additional Care

- If any tissue has been bitten off, bring it with the victim to the emergency room

Snakebites

Poisonous snakes in North America include rattlesnakes, copperheads, water moccasins (cottonmouths), coral snakes, and exotic species kept in captivity. Rattlesnake bites cause most snakebite deaths. Unless you are absolutely certain that a victim's snakebite was from a nonpoisonous snake, treat all snakebites as potentially dangerous. Antivenin is often available in areas where snakebites are common.

When You See

- Puncture marks in skin
- Complaint of pain or burning at bite site
- Redness and swelling
- *Depending on species:* difficulty breathing, numbness or muscle paralysis, nausea and vomiting, blurred vision, drowsiness or confusion, weakness

Do This First

1. Have the victim lie down and stay calm. (Do not move the victim unless absolutely necessary.) Keep the bitten area immobile and below the level of the heart.
2. Call 911.
3. Wash the bite wound with soap and water.
4. Remove jewelry or tight clothing before swelling begins.

Additional Care

- Do not try to catch the snake, but note its appearance and describe it to the healthcare provider
- Monitor the ABCs and give care as needed

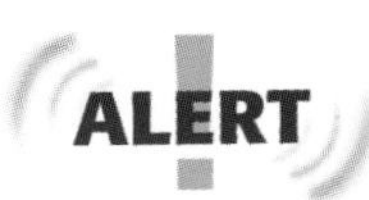

Snakebite

Do not put a tourniquet on the victim.
Do not cut the wound open to try to drain the venom out.
Do not try to suck out the venom.

Spider Bites

Many types of spiders bite, but only the venom of the black widow and brown recluse spider is serious and sometimes fatal (Figure 9-2). The black widow often has a red hourglass-shaped marking on the underside of the abdomen. The brown recluse has a violin-shaped marking on its back. An antivenin is available for black widow spider bites.

When You See

For black widow bite:

- Complaint of pain at bite site
- Red skin at site
- After 15 minutes to hours: sweating, nausea, stomach and muscle cramps, increased pain at site, dizziness or weakness, difficulty breathing

For brown recluse bite:

- Stinging sensation at site
- Over 8 to 48 hours: increasing pain, blistering at site, fever, chills, nausea or vomiting, joint pain, open sore at site

Do This First

1. If the victim has difficulty breathing, call 911. Call 911 immediately for a brown recluse spider bite. Monitor the ABCs and give care as needed.
2. Keep the bite area below the level of the heart.
3. Wash the area with soap and water.
4. Put ice or a cold pack on the bite area (Figure 9-3).

Additional Care

- Try to safely catch the spider to show the healthcare provider
- If 911 was not called the victim should go to the emergency room

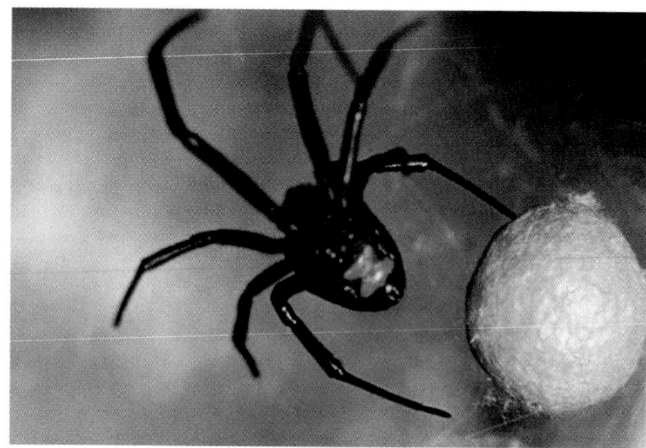

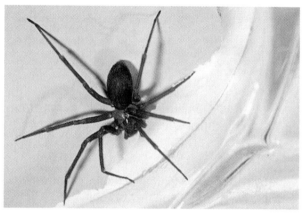

(a) Black widow spider

(b) Brown recluse spider

Figure 9-2 Poisonous spiders.

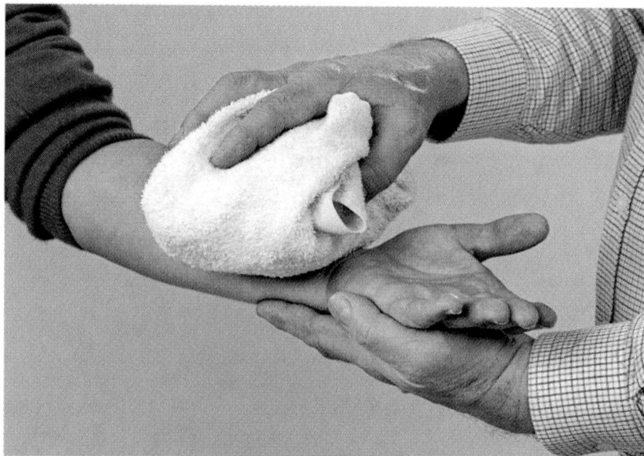

Figure 9-3 Put an ice or cold pack on a spider bite.

Tick Bites

Tick bites are not poisonous but can transmit serious diseases like Rocky Mountain spotted fever or Lyme disease. The tick embeds its mouth parts in the skin and may remain for days (Figure 9-4).

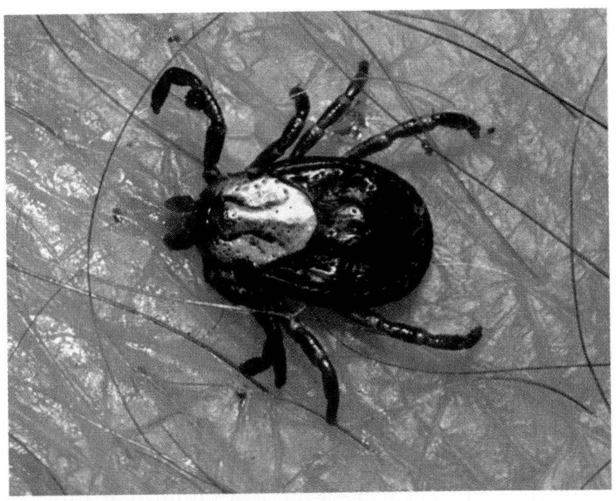

(a) Tick embedded in skin

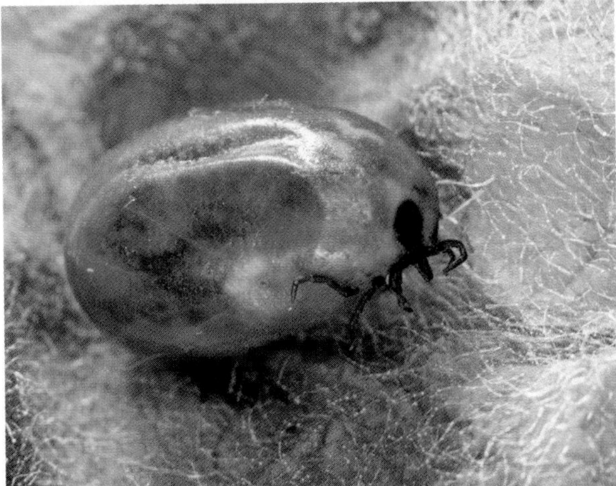

(b) Tick engorged

Figure 9-4 Tick bite.

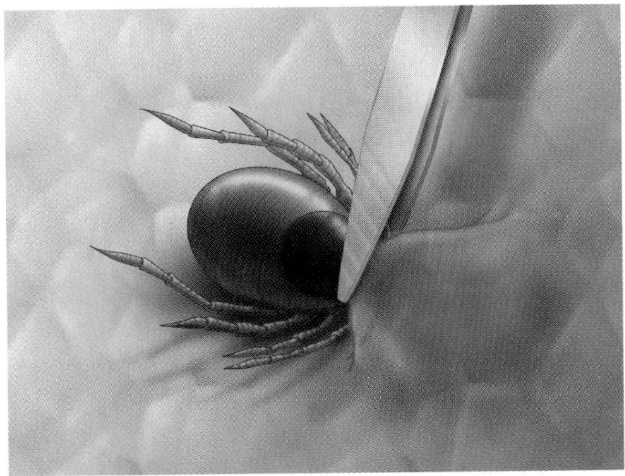

Figure 9-5 Grasp a tick close to the skin and pull very gently.

Additional Care

- Seek medical attention if a rash appears around the site or the victim later experiences fever, chills, joint pain, or other flu-like symptoms

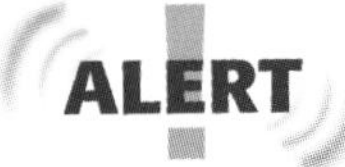

Tick Removal

Do not try to remove an embedded tick by covering it with petroleum jelly, soaking it with bleach, burning it away with a hot pin or other object, or similar methods. These methods may result in part of the tick remaining embedded in the skin.

When You See

- Tick embedded in skin

Do This First

1. Remove the tick by grasping it close to the skin with tweezers and pulling very gently until the tick finally lets go. Avoid pulling too hard or jerking, which may leave part of the tick in the skin (Figure 9-5).
2. Wash the area with soap and water.
3. Put an antiseptic such as rubbing alcohol on the site. Apply an antibiotic cream.

LYME DISEASE

Lyme disease, spread by ticks, has become a serious problem in many areas in the U.S. Lyme disease is a bacterial infectious disease that first causes fever, chills, and other flu-like symptoms and later on causes heart and neurological problems. Look for a bull's-eye rash that appears around the tick bite site 3 to 30 days later. Get medical attention if you have this rash or flu-like symptoms or joint pain after a tick bite.

To prevent tick bites:

- Keep lawns mowed, brush cleaned up, wood piles stacked off the ground

- Wear socks with shoes or boots. Tuck long pants into socks
- Light-colored clothing makes it easier to see ticks before they reach your skin
- Do not lay clothing, towels, etc. on the ground
- Comb or brush your hair after being in an infested area
- Check your body everywhere when bathing or showering

Bee and Wasp Stings

Bee, wasp, and other insect stings are not poisonous but can cause life-threatening allergic reactions in victims with severe allergies to them. (See Chapter 4.)

When You See

- Complaints of pain, burning, or itching at sting site
- Redness, swelling
- Stinger possibly still in skin

Do This First

1. Remove stinger from skin by scraping it away gently with a credit card or knife blade. Call 911 if victim has known allergy to stings.
2. Wash the area with soap and water.
3. Put ice or a cold pack on the sting site.
4. Watch victim for 30 minutes for any signs or symptoms of allergic reaction (difficulty breathing, swelling in other areas, anxiety, nausea, or vomiting); call 911 and treat for shock.

Additional Care

- An over-the-counter oral antihistamine may help reduce discomfort

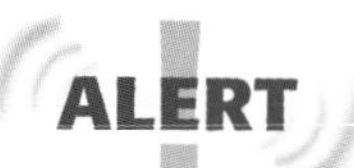

Insect Sting in Mouth

Have the victim suck on ice to reduce swelling. Call 911 if breathing becomes difficult.

Scorpion Stings

Scorpion stings are treated similarly to spider bites. Of the different types in the American Southwest, some are more poisonous than others and could be dangerous, especially for young children. Antivenin may be available in some areas (**Figure 9-6**).

When You See

- The scorpion sting with its tail
- Complaints of severe burning pain at sting site, later numbness, tingling
- Nausea, vomiting
- Difficulty swallowing
- Possible convulsions, coma

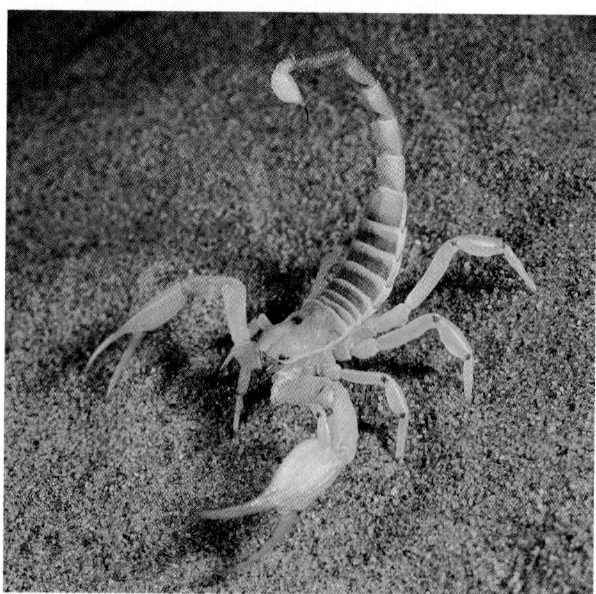

Figure 9-6 Scorpion.

Do This First

1. Call 911 if the victim is not breathing.
2. Monitor the ABCs and give care as needed.
3. Carefully wash the sting area.
4. Put ice or a cold pack on the area.
5. Seek urgent medical attention.

Additional Care

- Keep victim still

Learning Checkpoint 3

1. To minimize the risk of rabies from an animal bite, take which action?
   a. See a healthcare provider immediately
   b. See a healthcare provider if you experience heavy salivation 5 to 7 days after the bite
   c. Capture the animal and take it to a veterinarian for examination
   d. Soak the wound area with rubbing alcohol
2. Why can a human bite lead to a serious medical condition?

   ____

3. List three key actions to take for a victim of snakebite.

   ____

4. Check off situations in which you should call 911 for a spider bite:

   ____ a. All spider bites
   ____ b. Any spider bite in diabetic victim
   ____ c. Any brown recluse spider bite
   ____ d. If there is any pain at the bite site
   ____ e. If the victim has trouble breathing
   ____ f. If you have no ice to put on the bite

5. A tick is best removed from the skin using ____________.
6. A bee's stinger can be removed from the skin using ____________.
7. A coworker was stung by a honeybee when passing the flower garden by your building's entrance. As she tells you about this, you see that her face is turning red, the skin around her eyes and mouth looks puffy, and she seems short of breath. What are the most important actions to take first? Why?

   ____

Chapter 10

Heat and Cold Emergencies

CHAPTER PREVIEW

- Frostbite
- Hypothermia
- Heat Cramps
- Heat Exhaustion
- Heatstroke

Cold or hot environments can cause medical problems if the body is not protected from temperature extremes. Often cold- and heat-related injuries begin gradually, but if a person remains exposed to an extreme temperature, an emergency can develop. Untreated, it can lead to serious injury or death.

Cold Injuries

Exposure to cold temperatures can cause either localized freezing of skin and other tissues (**frostbite**) or lowering of the whole body's temperature (**hypothermia**). Frostbite occurs when the temperature is 32 degrees Fahrenheit or colder. Hypothermia can occur at much warmer temperatures if the body is unprotected, especially if the victim is wet, exposed a long time, or unable to restore body heat because of a medical condition.

Frostbite

Frostbite is the freezing of skin or deeper tissues. It usually happens to exposed skin areas on the head or face, hands, or feet. Wind chill increases the risk of frostbite. Severe frostbite kills tissue and can result in gangrene and having to amputate the body part (**Figure 10-1**).

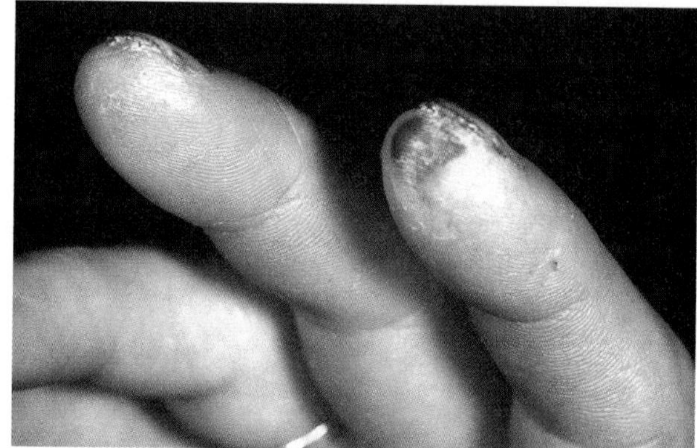

(a) Mild frostbite

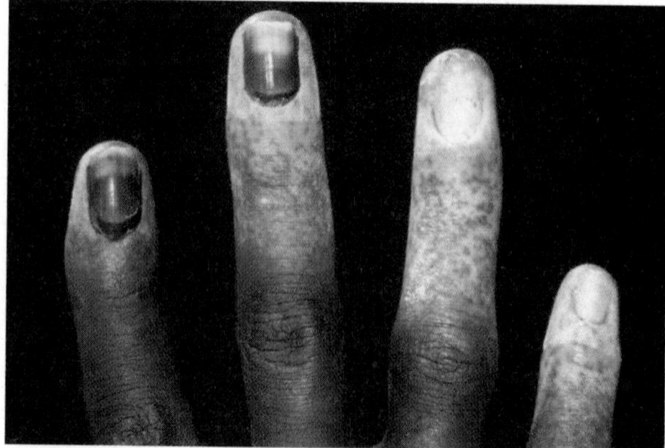

(b) Severe frostbite

Figure 10-1 Frostbite.

When You See

- Skin looks waxy and white, gray, yellow, or bluish
- The area is numb or feels tingly or aching

- Severe frostbite:
  - The area feels hard
  - May become painless
  - After warming, the area becomes swollen and may blister

Do This First

1. Move the victim to a warm environment. Hold the frostbitten area with your hands to warm it. (A victim with frostbitten hands can warm them in his or her armpits.) Check the victim also for hypothermia.
2. Remove any tight clothing or jewelry around the area.
3. Put dry gauze or fluffy cloth between frostbitten fingers or toes (Figure 10-2).
4. Seek medical attention as soon as possible.
5. Additionally for severe frostbite:
   a. Warm the frostbitten area in lukewarm, not hot, water for at least 20 minutes or up to 45 minutes (Figure 10-3).
   b. Protect the area from being touched or rubbed by clothing or objects.
   c. Elevate the area if possible to reduce swelling.

Additional Care

- The victim may choose to take aspirin (adults only), acetaminophen, or ibuprofen for pain
- Drink warm liquids *but not alcohol*
- Prevent the area from refreezing

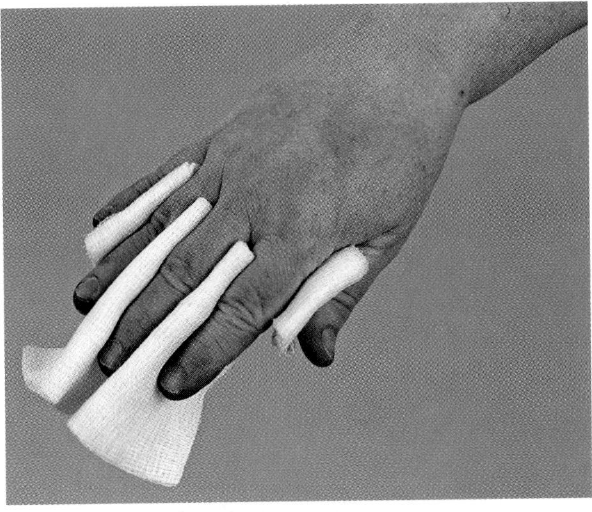

Figure 10-2 Protect between fingers and toes.

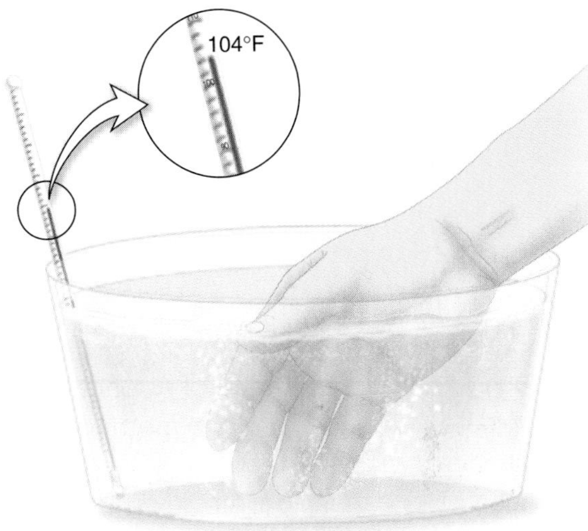

Figure 10-3 Warm the frostbitten area in lukewarm, not hot, water.

Learning Checkpoint 1

1. True or False: Rubbing frostbitten fingers is the best way to warm them.
2. Frostbitten skin usually has what color(s)?

   ____

3. A maintenance crewman comes into your building complaining of being very cold. He has lost his hat and his ears are white and hard and he says he has no feeling in them. Describe three actions to take for this man's frostbite.

   ____

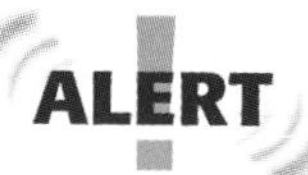

Frostbite

Do not rub frostbitten skin because this can damage the skin.
Do not rewarm frostbitten skin if it may be frozen again, which could worsen the injury.
Do not use a fire, heat lamp, hot water bottle, or heating pad to warm the area.
After rewarming, be careful not to break blisters.

Hypothermia

When the body cannot make heat as fast as it loses it in a cold environment, the person develops hypothermia. In hypothermia, the person's body temperature drops below 95 degrees Fahrenheit. Hypothermia can occur whenever and wherever a person feels cold, including indoors in poorly heated areas. It may occur gradually or quickly, especially with a wind chill or if the victim is wet.

FACTS ABOUT HYPOTHERMIA

- Hypothermia occurs more easily in elderly or ill people.
- People under the influence of alcohol or drugs are at greater risk for hypothermia.
- A person immersed in cold water cools 30 times faster than in cool air.
- Victims in cold water are more likely to die from hypothermia than to drown.
- Victims in cardiac arrest after immersion in cold water have been resuscitated after a long time underwater—don't give up!

When You See

- Shivering may be uncontrollable (but stops in severe hypothermia)
- Victim seems apathetic, confused, or irrational; may be belligerent
- Lethargy, clumsy movements, drowsiness
- Pale, cool skin–even under clothing
- Slow breathing
- Changing levels of responsiveness

Do This First

1. With an unresponsive victim, check the ABCs and provide care as needed. Call 911 for all severe hypothermia victims.
2. Quickly get the victim out of the cold, and remove any wet clothing.
3. Have the victim lie down, and cover him or her with blankets or warm clothing. (**Figure 10-4**).
4. Except in mild cases, the victim needs immediate medical care.

Additional Care

- Give an alert victim who can easily swallow warm drinks *but not alcohol*
- Stay with the victim until he or she reaches a healthcare provider or help arrives

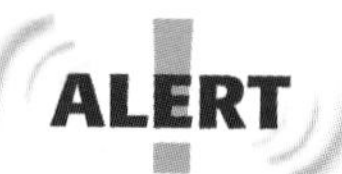

Hypothermia

Do not immerse a victim of hypothermia in hot water or use direct heat (hot water bottle, heat lamp, heating pad), because rapid warming can cause heart problems.

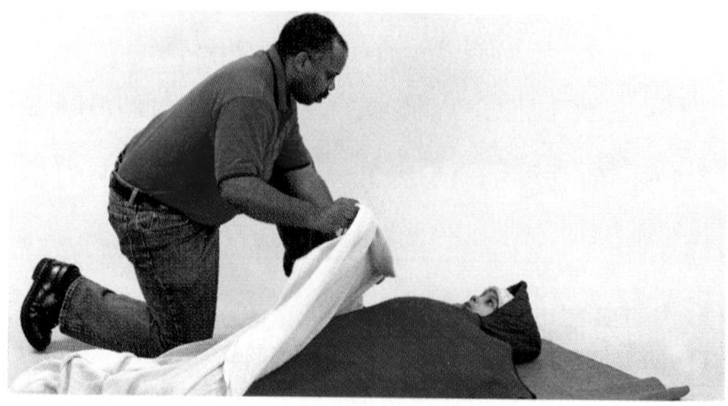

Figure 10-4 Warm a hypothermia victim with blankets, not with hot water.

Learning Checkpoint 2

1. True or False: Hypothermia occurs only when the air temperature is below freezing.

2. True or False: A hypothermia victim who is generating heat by shivering still needs first aid and warming.

3. A mildly hypothermic victim is brought into a ski lodge to be warmed. It will help to:

a. Give him a warm rum drink

b. Have him take off his outer clothes and sit close to the fire

c. Send him to a hot shower

d. Remove his damp clothing and warm him with a blanket

4. You are on a backpacking camping trip in the mountains and are caught in an unexpected snowstorm. On the way back down the mountain, about 4 miles from your car, you encounter a teenager sitting in the snow. His clothes are snowy and damp. He is lethargic and seems very confused. You call for help on your cell phone, but it will be at least 2 hours before the rescue team arrives. Using your usual camping gear, what first aid can you give this victim?

____

PREVENTING HYPOTHERMIA

When planning to be outdoors a long time, be prepared for a cold emergency.

Take along:

- Extra clothing, socks, sleeping bag or survival bag
- High-energy food bars, warm drinks
- No alcohol

Dress for the cold:

- Layer clothing
- Choose coat with wind- and waterproof outer layer
- Wear a hat (most body heat is lost from the head)

HEAT EMERGENCIES

Heat illnesses can result when people become overheated in a hot environment:

- ***Heat cramps*** are the least serious and usually first to occur.
- ***Heat exhaustion*** develops when the body becomes dehydrated in a hot environment.
- ***Heatstroke,*** with a seriously high body temperature, may develop from heat exhaustion. It is a medical emergency and, if untreated, usually causes death.

Heat Cramps

Activity in a hot environment may cause painful cramps in muscles, often in the lower legs or stomach muscles. Heat cramps may occur along with heat exhaustion and heatstroke.

When You See

- Signs of muscle pain, cramping, spasms
- Heavy sweating

Do This First

1. Have the person stop the activity and sit quietly in a cool place.

2. Give a sports drink or water.

Additional Care

- For abdominal cramps, continue resting in a comfortable position
- For leg cramps, stretch the muscle by extending the leg and flexing the ankle. Apply pressure to the cramped area.

Heat Exhaustion

Activity in a hot environment usually causes heavy sweating, which may lead to dehydration and depletion of salt and electrolytes in the body if the person does not get enough fluids. Unrelieved, heat exhaustion may develop into heatstroke, a true medical emergency.

When You See

- Heavy sweating
- Thirst
- Fatigue
- Heat cramps

Later signs and symptoms:

- Headache, dizziness
- Nausea, vomiting

Do This First

1. Move the victim from the heat to rest in a cool place. Loosen or remove unnecessary clothing.
2. Give a sports drink or water to drink.
3. Raise the feet 8–12 inches.
4. Cool the victim with one of these methods (Figure 10-5):
   - Put wet cloths on the forehead and body
   - Sponge the skin with cool water
   - Spray the skin with water from a spray bottle and then fan the area

Additional Care

- Seek medical care if the victim's condition worsens or does not improve within 30 minutes

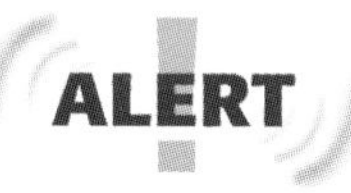

Heat Exhaustion

Do not give a heat exhaustion or heatstroke victim salt tablets. Use a sports drink instead (if the victim is awake and alert). Do not give liquids containing caffeine or alcohol. If the victim is lethargic, nauseous, or vomiting, do not give any liquids.

Learning Checkpoint 3

1. True or False: For abdominal heat cramps, the best care is vigorous massage and stomach kneading.
2. To treat heat cramps:
   a. Immerse the victim in a bathtub of cold water
   b. Give a sports drink or water to drink
   c. Keep the victim very active until the cramp works itself out
   d. Do not let the victim eat or drink anything
3. Heat cramps can also occur with heat __________ and heat __________.

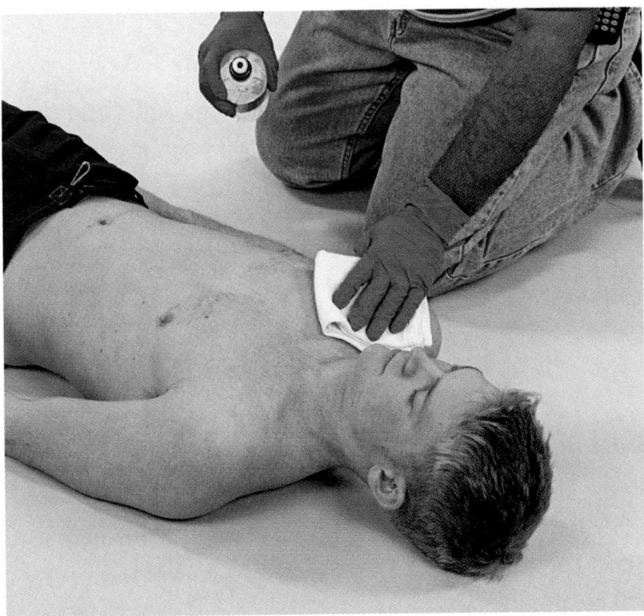

Figure 10-5 Cool a victim with heat exhaustion.

Learning Checkpoint 4

1. True or False: Give salt tablets to victims who have both heat cramps and heat exhaustion.
2. The problem of heat exhaustion begins when a person in a hot environment is not getting enough ________.
3. List three possible ways to cool a victim with heat exhaustion.

   ____

4. On a hot day you are called to your company's loading dock, where a workman who has been unloading trucks is sitting on the pavement in the sun. He is sweating heavily and says he has a headache and feels nauseous. Someone has already given him a sports drink. What should you do now? List in correct order the first four actions you would take.

   ____

Heatstroke

Heatstroke is a life-threatening emergency that is more common during hot summer periods. It may develop slowly over several days or more rapidly when engaged in strenuous activity in the heat. The victim may be dehydrated and not sweating when heatstroke gradually develops, or may be sweating heavily from exertion. Heatstroke causes a body temperature of 104 degrees Fahrenheit or higher and is different from heat exhaustion:

- In heatstroke the victim's skin is flushed and feels very hot to the touch; in heat exhaustion the skin may be pale and clammy
- In heatstroke the victim becomes very confused and irrational and may become unresponsive or have convulsions; in heat exhaustion the victim is dizzy or disoriented

When You See

- Skin flushed and very hot to the touch, sweating may have stopped
- Fast breathing
- Headache, dizziness, extreme confusion
- Irrational behavior
- Possible convulsions or unresponsiveness

Do This First

1. Call 911.
2. Move the victim to a cool place.
3. Remove outer clothing.
4. Cool the victim quickly with any means at hand:
    - Wrap the victim in a wet sheet and keep it wet
    - Sponge the victim with cold water
    - Spray the skin with water from a spray bottle and then fan the area
    - Put ice bags or cool packs beside the neck, armpits, and groin
5. Keep cooling until the victim's temperature drops to approximately 100 degrees Fahrenheit.

Additional Care

- Monitor the ABCs and provide care as needed
- Put an unresponsive victim in the recovery position
- Protect a victim having convulsions from injury (see Chapter 8)

PREVENTING HEAT EMERGENCIES

- In hot environments wear loose, lightweight clothing
- Rest frequently in shady or cool areas
- Drink adequate fluids
- Avoid exertion if overweight or elderly

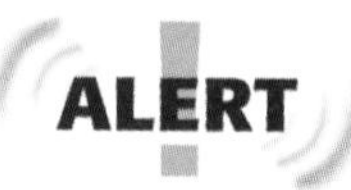

Heatstroke

The victim should not take pain relievers or salt tablets.
Do not give any beverage containing caffeine or alcohol.
If the victim is nauseous or vomiting, do not give liquids.

Learning Checkpoint 5

1. True or False: It is safe to drive a heatstroke victim home after you have given first aid to cool his or her body down to 100 degrees Fahrenheit, as long as the victim is feeling better.

2. In what situation should you call 911 for a heatstroke victim?

____

3. Describe how a heatstroke victim's behavior may be different from how that person usually behaves.

____

4. Your company's annual picnic and softball game happens to fall on the hottest day of the year. Your supervisor knows you have first aid training and asks you to help out to make sure none of the company "athletes" has problems with heat exhaustion or heatstroke.

a. To be prepared for these possibilities, what things should you make sure are present at the picnic/ballfield site?

____

b. You decide to give a safety pep talk to the teams before the game begins. What would you tell them about how to prevent heat emergencies? What signs and symptoms of a potential problem should players watch out for in others on their team?

____

c. Despite these precautions, by the seventh inning your center fielder seems to be showing signs and symptoms of heatstroke. What is the first step you should take?

____

Chapter

11 Rescuing and Moving Victims

CHAPTER PREVIEW

Before you can check the ABCs and give first aid, you have to reach the victim. Sometimes the scene is dangerous and you must stay away or take special precautions. Sometimes there is more than one victim and you have to decide whom to care for first. Sometimes the victim must be moved, if it is safe to do so, before you can give first aid.

Rescuing a Victim

Three common situations involving victim rescue are fires, hazardous materials incidents, and motor vehicle crashes when the vehicle is on fire.

Fire

When You See

- Flames or smoke
- A fire alarm sounding

Do This First

1. Remove everyone from the area. Close doors behind you as you leave.
2. Call 911, set off alarms, or follow other workplace protocols.
3. Use a fire extinguisher to combat a fire only if:
   - The fire is small
   - You can easily and quickly escape the area
   - You know how to use the fire extinguisher
   - You can stay between the exit and the fire, so that you can always safely get out
4. Do not enter an area of flames and smoke in an attempt to rescue others.
5. If trapped inside:
   - In a smoky room crawl along the floor where there is breathable air
   - Do not open a door that feels hot
   - Do not use elevators
   - If stuck inside, turn off the ventilation system, stuff towels or rags (wet if possible) in door cracks and vents, and use a phone to report your location

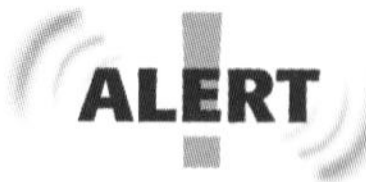

Victim Rescue

Never put yourself at risk to rescue a victim. When hazards are present, leave the rescue to the professionals. Do not try to perform any rescue technique you have not been trained to do. If you are injured when trying to rescue a victim, the professionals will then have two victims to rescue and treat.

PREVENTING FIRES

Workplace fires and explosions kill 200 workers a year. OSHA has many requirements for fire prevention in workplaces.

Key guidelines for fire prevention:

- Employees should be trained what to do in a fire and how to evacuate
- Emergency fire exits must be present, not blocked, and properly marked with signs
- If portable fire extinguishers are present, employees must be trained to use them
- Flammable and combustible materials must be stored properly and safely
- An emergency evacuation plan is required for employees with disabilities
- Many work sites must have additional safety controls including emergency action plans, fixed fire extinguishing systems, alarm systems, hazardous materials procedures, and other controls. Know what OSHA standards apply in your workplace.

In the home and other settings:

- Have smoke detectors in appropriate locations and replace batteries twice a year; check frequently that detectors are functioning
- Plan and practice a fire escape route. Be sure children can follow the plan.
- Keep a fire extinguisher in the kitchen
- Keep curtains and clothing away from fireplaces, stoves, and space heaters
- Do not overload electrical sockets. Replace frayed or damaged electrical cords.
- Eliminate fire hazards such as rags soaked with combustible paints or chemicals
- Keep matches and flammables away from children

Hazardous Materials

Treat any unknown substance as a hazard until proven otherwise. Avoid any spilled liquid or powder as well as possible vapors. Because the cleanup of hazardous materials takes special training, knowledge, and equipment, leave this to "hazmat" professionals.

When You See

- Warning signs or placards (with "flammable" or other warning terms) (Figure 11-1)
- Any spilled substance
- Vapors you can see or fumes you can smell

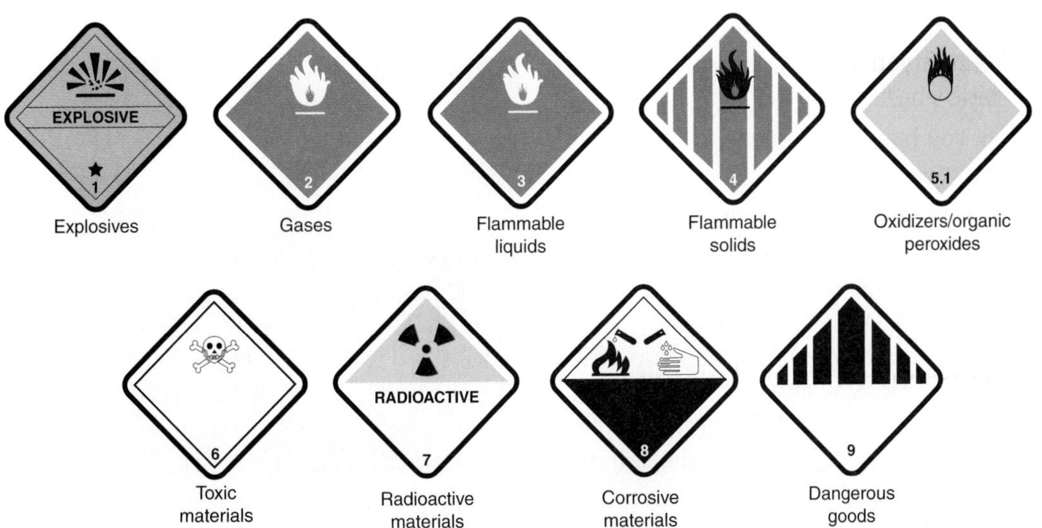

Figure 11-1 A variety of hazardous materials placards.

Do This First

1. Stay out of the area and keep bystanders away.
2. Outside, stay upwind of the area to avoid possible fumes.
3. Call 911.
4. Approach the victim only if you are sure it is safe to do so. With a large exposure to hazardous materials, guide the victim to an emergency shower. Do only what you have been trained to do.

Additional Care

- If safe to do so, give first aid for a chemical burn or smoke inhalation (see Chapter 5)

Vehicle Crashes

Vehicle crash scenes can be extremely dangerous for rescuers because of the risks of passing traffic, fire, vehicle instability, and other factors. Rescuers have been injured by accidentally setting off an automatic airbag when attempting to reach a victim. For all these reasons it is crucial to ensure the scene is safe before approaching the vehicle and providing care for the victim.

When You See

- A victim inside a motor vehicle after a crash

Do This First

1. Stop a safe distance past the crash and turn on your vehicle's hazard lights.
2. Call 911 if you have a cell phone, or ask someone else to call.
3. If available, set up warning triangles well back from the scene to warn oncoming traffic. Flares should be used only when there are no spilled chemicals and no chance of grass fire.
4. Ensure the scene is safe before you approach the crashed vehicle. Stay away if there are risks from passing traffic, downed electrical wires, fire, vehicle instability, etc. Do not try to stabilize the vehicle unless you have special training.
5. Do not try to remove a victim trapped inside a vehicle; wait for professional rescuers.
6. Assume that an unresponsive victim may have a neck injury. If the scene is safe support the victim's head and neck with your hands (**Figure 11-2**).
7. Do not move the victim unless there is an immediate threat of fire. If so, get several bystanders to help to move the victim while you support the victim's head in line with the body the whole time.
8. Monitor the ABCs and care for any serious injuries while waiting for help.

Multiple Victims

An incident may involve multiple victims who need first aid care. In such a case the first thing you must do is decide who needs your care most and who can wait until others can help. This process of setting priorities is called **triage** (**Figure 11-3**).

Triage systems usually put each victim in one of four categories:

- ***1st priority (critical condition):*** victims with life-threatening injuries who cannot wait for help
- ***2nd priority (serious condition):*** victims with injuries that need care very soon but may be able to wait for help

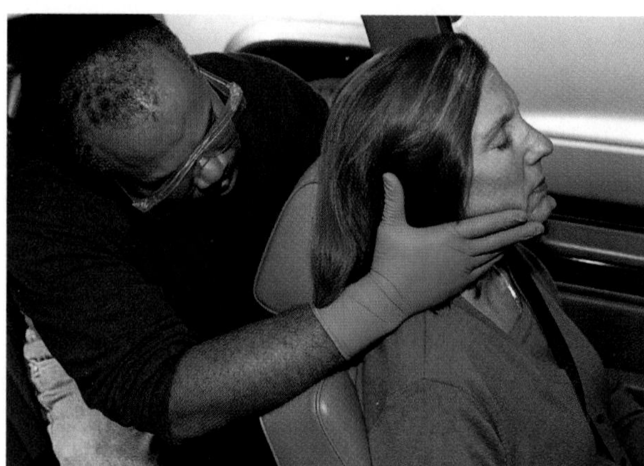

Figure 11-2 If a spinal injury is likely, support the head and neck with your hands.

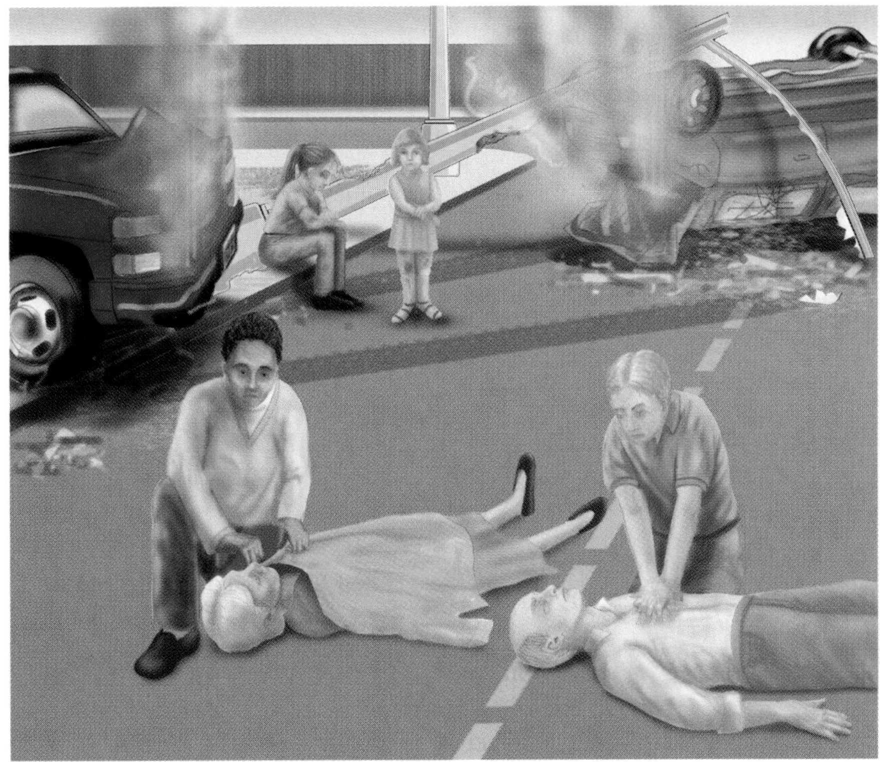

Figure 11-3 In an emergency with multiple victims, first determine which are highest priority for first aid.

Learning Checkpoint 1

1. With a fire the ***first*** action to take is:

a. Get everyone out and call 911

b. Throw water on the fire immediately

c. Use a fire extinguisher

d. Close all doors and windows

2. If you are caught in a building on fire:

a. Stay low to the floor

b. Feel doors before opening them

c. Use stairs, not the elevator

d. All of the above

3. True or False: OSHA requires fire prevention and safety guidelines in the workplace.

4. True or False: The first action to take with a spilled dry chemical is to vacuum it up.

5. True or False: Spilled liquids may produce poisonous vapors.

6. You are the first on the scene where a car has crashed into a telephone pole. After you ensure the scene is safe, you approach the car and find the driver alone, slumped forward against the steering wheel unresponsive. What can you do to help?

____

- *3rd priority (stable condition):* those with minor injuries, who can walk.
- *4th priority (obviously dead or dying):* those who cannot be saved.

When You See

- Two or more victims needing care
- A situation (such as an explosion or multi-vehicle crash) in which multiple victims are likely to be found

Do This First

1. Call 911 immediately. Tell the dispatcher there are multiple victims.
2. Ask any victims who can walk (3rd priority) to move to one side. These victims do not have immediately life-threatening problems.
3. With remaining victims, starting with unresponsive victims, quickly check the ABCs of each, looking for life-threatening injuries (1st priority). Spend a minute or less with each victim and do not start giving care until you have checked all victims.
4. Care for 1st priority victims first. Move to 2nd priority victims only when the 1st priority victims are stable. Ask any bystanders with first aid training to help you with other victims.
5. When help arrives, quickly tell the EMS professionals about the victims present. Offer to help them care for victims.

Moving Victims

Moving an injured victim is more likely to cause further injury than not. Wait for the professionals who have training and equipment to transport the victim to advanced medical care.

When You See

Consider moving a victim only if:

- Fire or explosion is likely
- Poisonous vapors are present
- The structure is collapsing
- The victim needs to be moved into position for life-saving care
- The victim is in the way of another seriously injured victim

Do This First

1. Try to move the victim only if you are physically able and can do it safely.
2. Get help from others at the scene.

Learning Checkpoint 2

1. True or False: A victim with a broken arm is a 2nd priority in a multiple-victim incident.
2. True or False: Victims with life-threatening injuries are 1st priority in a multiple-victim incident.
3. You arrive alone at a construction site where a collapsed wall has injured four workers. Using standard triage priorities, rank these four in terms of who gets care first, second, third, and fourth:

   ______ **a.** A woman with a bruised face and abrasions on her arms, who is walking around holding her bleeding forehead

   ______ **b.** A man on the ground with no apparent external injuries but who is unresponsive

   ______ **c.** A man who is not breathing, whose chest has caved in under a steel beam, and who is surrounded by a pool of blood

   ______ **d.** A man sitting leaning against the rubble, looking very pale, who says he feels nauseous.

3. With an unresponsive victim or a victim with a spinal injury, support the head and neck in line with the body during the move.
4. Use good body mechanics: bend at your knees and hips (not your back), lift with your legs (not your back), take short steps, and move forward rather than backward.
5. If alone, the easiest emergency move is a drag:
   - Use the shoulder drag (supporting the victim's head) or ankle drag for short distances
   - Use the blanket drag to support the victim's head for a longer distance
6. With the help of one or more others:
   - Use the two-person assist or two-handed seat carry for a responsive victim
   - Use three to six rescuers with the hammock carry for an unresponsive victim

Moving a Victim

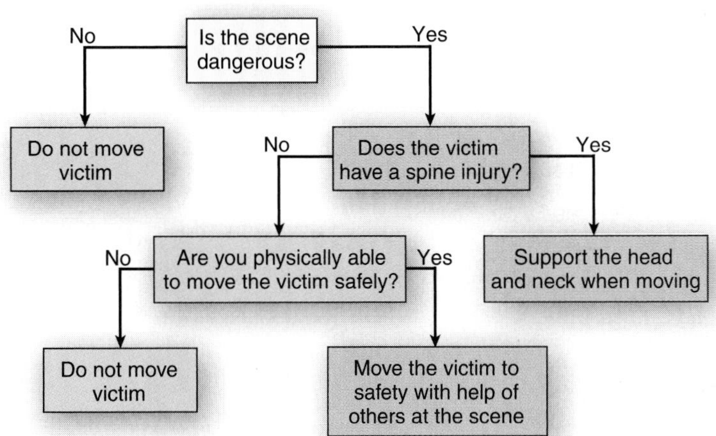

Learning Checkpoint 3

1. Check situations in which you should consider moving a victim:

_____ **a.** Fire is present

_____ **b.** Freezing cold environment

_____ **c.** Small child with severe burns

_____ **d.** A victim going into shock

_____ **e.** Bleeding victim inside a car

_____ **f.** Strong smell of natural gas in the room

_____ **g.** The hospital is only a short drive

_____ **h.** One victim is lying on top of another

2. If you have to move an unresponsive injured victim by yourself, an effective method would be:

a. Sling the victim over your shoulder

b. Cradle the victim in your arms

c. Grab both the victim's wrists and pull him or her along

d. Use a blanket drag to support the victim's head

Perform the Skill

Moving Victims

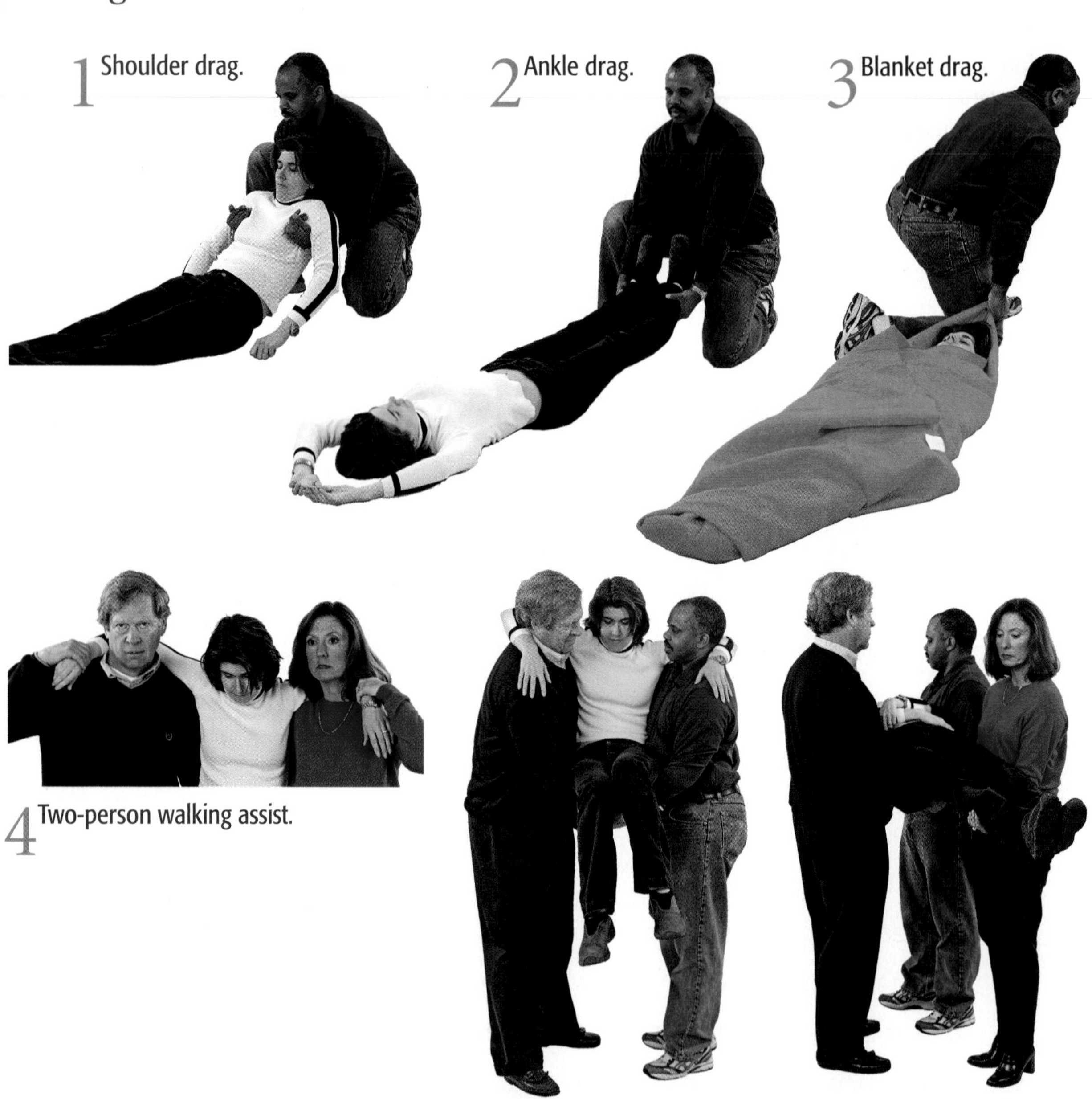

1 Shoulder drag.

2 Ankle drag.

3 Blanket drag.

4 Two-person walking assist.

5 Two-handed seat carry.

6 Hammock carry with multiple rescuers.

Appendix

A Summary of Basic Life Support

Step	Infant (under 1 year)	Child (1–8 years)	Adult (over 8 years)
1. Check for responsiveness	Stimulate to check response	"Are you okay" Tap shoulder	"Are you okay" Tap shoulder
2. If unresponsive, call 911	Send someone to call Give 1 minute of care before calling yourself if alone	Send someone to call Give 1 minute of care before calling yourself if alone (except for known heart problem)	Send someone to call if alone Call immediately (give 1 minute of care for victim of drowning, poisoning, injury)
3. If unresponsive: Open airway	Head tilt-chin lift (but do not overextend neck)	Head tilt-chin lift or jaw thrust	Head tilt-chin lift or jaw thrust
4. Check breathing	Look, listen, feel for breathing	Look, listen, feel for breathing	Look, listen, feel for breathing
5. If not breathing: Give 2 breaths, watch chest rise	Use barrier device or cover mouth/nose or nose Each breath lasts 1 to 1½ seconds	Use barrier device or cover mouth, or nose Each breath lasts 1 to 1½ seconds	Use barrier device or cover mouth, nose, or stoma Each breath lasts 2 seconds
6. If chest does not rise: Reposition airway and try 2 breaths again	Each breath lasts 1 to 1½ seconds	Each breath lasts 1 to 1½ seconds	Each breath lasts 2 seconds

(continued)

Step	Infant (under 1 year)	Child (1–8 years)	Adult (over 8 years)
7. If chest still does not rise: Start CPR for airway obstruction (choking care)	For compressions use 2 fingers one finger-width below line between nipples Compress chest ½–1 inch Compress at rate of at least 100/minute 5 compressions per 1 breath	For compressions use one hand midway between nipples Compress chest 1–1½ inches Compress at rate of 100/minute 5 compressions per 1 breath	For compressions use both hands, one on top of other, midway between nipples Compress chest 1½–2 inches Compress at rate of 100/minute 15 compressions per 2 breaths
8. Check for signs of circulation	Scan body for movement, breathing, coughing, and normal skin condition	Scan body for movement, breathing, coughing, and normal skin condition	Scan body for movement, breathing, coughing, and normal skin condition
9. If circulation signs present but no breathing, give rescue breathing	1 breath every 3 seconds	1 breath every 3 seconds	1 breath every 5 seconds
10. If no signs of circulation present, continue CPR	Cycles of 5 compressions and 1 breath	Cycles of 5 compressions and 1 breath	Cycles of 15 compressions and 2 breaths
11. Continue to check for breathing and signs of circulation	Look, listen, and feel for breathing and scan body for signs of circulation	Look, listen, and feel for breathing and scan body for signs of circulation	Look, listen, and feel for breathing and scan body for signs of circulation
12. Use AED when available (if no breathing or signs of circulation)	Do not use AED	Use only pediatric electrode pads	Use adult AED electrode pads
13. If victim recovers breathing and signs of circulation, put in recovery position	Hold infant and monitor ABCs	Lay on side in recovery position and monitor ABCs	Lay on side in recovery position and monitor ABCs

Index

S

T

U

W